Fauci versus Duesberg

The battle about AIDS that brought Chronic Fatigue Syndrome out of the closet

Two chapters from *The Chronic Fatigue Syndrome Epidemic Cover-up Volume Two*

Charles Ortleb

Published by HHV-6 University, Salem, Massachusetts

Distributed by Rubicon Media

PRINTED IN THE UNITED STATES OF AMERICA

ISBN: 9798649198189

10 9 8 7 6 5 4 3 2 1
First Edition

Fauci

The Bernie Madoff of Science and the HIV Ponzi
Scheme that Concealed the Chronic Fatigue
Syndrome Epidemic

Introduction

This little book consists of two chapters about Anthony Fauci and Peter Duesberg from *The Chronic Fatigue Epidemic Cover-up Volume Two.*

*

If justice and truth prevail in the world, one day what has been called "AIDS" will be renamed "Holocaust II." While gay people were secondary victims of what is referred to as "The Holocaust," or "Holocaust I," they were the main attraction in "Holocaust II." The heterosexist motivation of their stigmatization and persecution in both holocausts were similar even if the manner in which they were harmed was different. I have used the term "Iatrogenocide" to describe what happened to gay men (and others) during Holocaust II.

I was a witness to the AIDS epidemic from the very beginning. As the publisher and editor-in-chief of *New York Native,* I inadvertently oversaw the reporting of the very first story about the epidemic. After hearing about a strange pneumonia occurring in gay men in New York City, I asked a physician to make inquiries with the public health authorities. In a story headlined "Disease Rumors Largely Unfounded" published in our May 18, 1981 issue, Dr. Lawrence Mass wrote, "Last week there were rumors that an exotic new disease had hit the gay community in New York. Here are the facts. From the New York City Department of Health, Dr. Steve Phillips explained that the rumors are for the most part unfounded. Each year, approximately 12 to 24 cases of infection with a protozoa-like organism, Pneumocystis carinii, are reported in the New York City area. The organism is not exotic; in fact, it's ubiquitous. But most of us have a natural or easily acquired immunity."

Six weeks later it turned out that the rumors were true when the CDC reported on the first cases of what would be called AIDS. It is hard to overstate the shock and terror that gripped the gay community in New York City and eventually around the world. People dreaded waking up each morning as bad news just got worse and worse. Given that my paper seemed to be at the ground zero of the event, I made the conscious decision to devote *New York Native* to covering every detail of the story. For the first two years our coverage was so thorough that some people started referring to my newspaper as "The New York Native Journal of Medicine." Many of our readers and advertisers resented our coverage and wanted us to focus on positive stories. But I felt that we had a responsibility get to the bottom of what was going on.

As the cases mounted and the gay community began to accept the reality of the epidemic, our coverage began to be appreciated and *New York Native* became a trusted source for the latest news about AIDS. In the April 25, 1985 issue of *Rolling Stone*, David Black said that *New York Native* deserved a Pulitzer Prize for our reporting. In his bestselling book, *And the Band Played On*, Randy Shilts wrote, "Because of the extraordinary reporting of the *New York Native*, the city's gay community had been exposed to far more information about AIDS than San Francisco in 1981 and 1982." And in the March 23, 1989 *Rolling Stone*, Katie Leishman wrote, "It is undeniable that many major AIDS stories were Ortleb's months and sometimes years before mainstream journalists too them up." But that love affair with *New York Native* was about to end abruptly.

As I have detailed in my history of *New York Native*, *The Chronic Fatigue Syndrome Epidemic Cover-up*, as the epidemic went on and our reporting became more investigative, I began to notice serious credibility gaps in what the Centers for Disease Control was telling the public about the AIDS epidemic. AIDS increasingly reminded me of the period of egregious government mendacity that occurred during the Vietnam era. As the government began to build a paradigm around the notion that AIDS was caused by a retrovirus ultimately labelled "HIV," I watched as credible critics of the retroviral theory were silenced and vilified. I discuss the heroic voices that spoke out in *Peter Duesberg and the Duesbergians*.

My newspaper became even more controversial when we began reporting on another epidemic called Chronic Fatigue Syndrome.

From our extensive reporting, it was hard not to conclude that Chronic Fatigue Syndrome is part of the AIDS epidemic and is linked to AIDS by a virus called HHV-6 which government scientists refused to take seriously.

As AIDS activists increasing lined up behind the government's HIV/AIDS paradigm and draconian public health agenda, the inconvenient truths my newspaper was reporting about HHV-6 and Chronic Fatigue Syndrome became increasingly unpopular. Nobody wanted to believe that the elite AIDS doctors and scientists might have gotten AIDS totally wrong. Act Up, New York's powerful AIDS activist group, voted to boycott *New York Native* and they did anything they could to put us out of business. Finally, in January 1997, we published our final issue.

In the last twenty years, I have given a great deal of thought to the nature of what happened to my newspaper and to the integrity of AIDS science and medicine. A number of my thoughts on the subject are collected in *Iatrogenocide: Notes for a Political Philosophy of Epidemiology and Science.* I have also written a play about the politics of the epidemic called *The Black Party.* My thoughts about the racial politics of AIDS can be found in a novella, *The Closing Argument.*

I have come to the conclusion that the similarities between AIDS science and Nazi science are too obvious for people of conscience to ignore. In his groundbreaking book about Nazi treatment of Jews, *"Life Unworthy of Life": Racial Phobia and Mass Murder in Hitler's Germany,* James M. Glass writes, "It was not cultural propagandists who organized the infamous 'special treatment' of the Jews; it was the public health officials, the scientific journals, the physicians, the administrators, and the lawyers, who feared the very presence of the Jews would endanger their families, their bodies, and ultimately their lives. To think of the Jew in such terms is insane from our perspective, but it was held to be sane in the culture caught up in the phobic projection of infection onto the Jews and the scientific authority legitimizing such beliefs." In many ways AIDS, or what I call "Holocaust II," involved what could be called "special epidemiological treatment" of the gays which was created and supported by health officials, scientific journals, physicians, administrators, lawyers, activists, celebrities, and many others. While the manner in which AIDS is understood by public health authorities and the general public is assumed to be sane, a closer look reveals that a genocidal insanity lurks beneath the surface. In the case of AIDS, a fraudulent and phobic epidemiology has been used to scapegoat and biomedically persecute the gay community. And many others.

In this chapter from The Chronic Fatigue Syndrome Epidemic Cover-up Volume Two, I discuss the scientist I consider to be among the important "architects" of Holocaust II. He played a key role in creating the kind of science which I describe in *Iatrogenocide* as being abnormal, totalitarian, and sociopathic.

I believe that when honest and brave scientists finally give Fauci's AIDS and Chronic Fatigue Syndrome work the due diligence it deserves, they will recognize that he has essentially been running a scientific Ponzi scheme for decades. Science now has its own Bernie Madoff.

Chronic Fatigue Syndrome and the HIV Ponzi Scheme

November 2, 1984 was an especially tragic day in the Chronic Fatigue Syndrome/AIDS epidemic. That was the day Anthony Fauci became the Director of the National Institutes of Allergy and Infectious Diseases. (NIAID). (*Good Intentions* p.128) It was the day a thin-skinned, physically ultra-diminutive man with a legendary Napoleonic attitude was positioned by destiny to become the de facto AIDS Czar. In the fog of culpability that constitutes what could be called "Holocaust II" one thing is clear: the buck, on its way to the very top of the government, at least pauses at the megalomaniac desk of Anthony Fauci.

In his book, *Good Intentions*, Bruce Nussbaum writes, "Fauci looked as if he had just stepped out of a limousine. Trim and athletic, Fauci's tailored suits, cuff-linked shirts, and aviator glasses set him far apart from the rest of the scientists and administrators at the NIH." (*GI* p.128) Fauci had risen quickly at NIH. According to Nussbaum, he began work at NIH in 1968 after his residency and "by 1977 he was deputy clinical director of NIAID." (*GI* p.128) Nussbaum describes Fauci as "an aggressive administrator," not a "details man," "a big picture kind of guy." (GI p.128) Nussbaum reports that "Fauci saw AIDS as a dreadful disease—and an opportunity for NIAID to grow into a much bigger, more powerful institute. AIDS was his big chance. He wasn't known as a brilliant scientist, and he had little background in managing a big bureaucracy; but Fauci did have ambition and drive to spare. This lackluster scientist was about to find his true vocation—empire building." (*GI* p.128) Unfortunately, the empire his extreme ambition would build was "Holocaust II." If the mantra during Watergate was "follow the money," the mantra for uncovering the crimes of "Holocaust II" (other than "follow the heterosexism") could be "follow the empire building." And one of the morals of the story is that "lackluster" can have extreme consequences.

According to Nussbaum, in order to make his dreams come true, Fauci had to fight "for a bigger piece of the AIDS research pie" which he succeeded at by getting a sizable amount of the funds that Congress appropriated for AIDS research. (*GI* p.129) Fauci also had to fight to get AIDS out of the claws of the National Cancer Institute where the virus that was believed to be the cause of AIDS had been discovered (or, more accurately, stolen). Fauci argued that it was his institute's right to take on the lion's share of the research because, although AIDS did involve cancer (Kaposi's sarcoma), it was, after all, an infectious disease. Fauci got his way and his success is reflected in the evolving financial numbers Nussbaum provides: "A growing budget for AIDS research, like a rising tide, lifted Tony Fauci's profile considerably on the NIH campus. In 1982, NIAID received $297,000 in AIDS funding. In 1986 it received $63 million. In 1987, the sum reached $146 million. By 1990, NIAID's annual AIDS funding was pushing half a billion dollars. Tony Fauci's ship had come in." (*GI* p.132)

Fauci's ship coming in meant the gay community's would be sinking fast. It would fall to Anthony Fauci to be the Enforcer-in-Chief of the "homodemiological" HIV/AIDS and "Chronic Fatigue Syndrome is not AIDS" paradigms of "Holocaust II." No one can argue that he didn't do a spectacular job of paradigm enforcement for three dreadful decades.

Starting in the mid-1980s, an organization called the American Foundation for AIDS Research (amfAR) played a multifaceted role of raising money for HIV research and enlisting celebrities in a glamorous and ultimately shameful HIV propaganda campaign that made the putatively private organization essentially a de facto arm of the government's HIV/AIDS establishment. If one considers the HIV theory of AIDS a Potemkin biomedical village that gays were forced to live in, then amfAR is one of its leading real estate agents. John Lauritsen, in his book, *The AIDS War*, writes that "[amfAR] was founded as an alternative to the AIDS establishment, to provide funding for research that was *not* predicated on the 'AIDS virus' hypothesis. It didn't last long. . . . I am not aware that even a penny has ever been given to a researcher who publicly expressed doubts as to the etiological role of HIV or the benefits of the nucleoside analogues." (*AW* p.437)

In addition to becoming one of the leading private promoters of the government's HIV/AIDS paradigm propaganda, amfAR played a disturbing role in squelching serious scientific criticism of the HIV hypothesis and in helping turn the entire field of AIDS into a world of heterosexist, totalitarian, and abnormal science. Lauritsen describes an historically important amfAR moment in the AIDS disaster in his first book *Poison by Prescription*: "A 'Scientific Forum on the Etiology of AIDS,' sponsored by the American Foundation for AIDS Research (amfAR), was held on 9 April 1988 at the George Washington University in Washington, D.C. In the words of the amfAR 'fact sheet', the forum was convened to critically examine the evidence that human immunodeficiency virus (HIV) or other agents give rise to the disease complex known as AIDS." (*PBP* p.143)

According to Lauritsen, it was supposedly an opportunity for Peter Duesberg, the University of California at Berkeley retrovirologist who first challenged the HIV theory of AIDS "to confront members of the 'AIDS Establishment' over their hypothesis." (*PBP* p.143) He reports, however, that "Despite these praiseworthy intentions, the forum appears to have had a hidden agenda; to discredit Duesberg." (*PBP* p.143) Lauritsen characterized the forum as a "Kangaroo Court." The forum would make a great scene in a play about the nasty, zany world of AIDS and HIV pseudoscience. It was anything but an honest, open collegial discussion about the nature of AIDS. Scientific philosopher Thomas Kuhn Kuhn would roll over in his grave if anyone called it genuinely scientific. By Kuhn's standards, some of the leading voices at the forum may have even demonstrated that they should not even have been considered real scientists. Politicians, yes, scientists not so much. Even the HIV theory's ardent acolyte, Michael Specter, the reporter from *The Washington Post* (and future *New Yorker* writer) who was among the 17 journalists at the Forum, saw through the charade, noting that the meeting "was billed as a scientific forum on the cause of AIDS but was really an attempt to put Duesberg's theories to rest." (*PBP* p.144) It was more like they wanted to put Duesberg himself permanently to rest.

The meeting had the tone and style that was endemic to HIV/AIDS research and characteristic of abnormal and totalitarian science. Lauritsen reported that "While no blows were struck, some of the HIV protagonists fell below the standards of civility that are expected in scholarly debate . . . . At all times Duesberg retained good manners and a sense of humor, in the face of invective, insults, and clowning from his opponents." (*PBP* p.144)

One of the signs that AIDS in general was being conducted in the opposite world of what could be called abnormal, totalitarian science was the uncanny willingness of the scientists to abandon the traditional rules of evidence known as Koch's postulates. Instead, AIDS researchers, including the ones at the amfAR forum, were willing to "revise Koch's in a more permissive direction: it would no longer be necessary to find the microbe in all cases of the disease. Mere correlations between microbial *antibodies* and the progression of the disease would be sufficient. HIV could be proved 'epidemiologically' to be the cause of AIDS." (*PBP* p.145) Given the unrecognized sexual politics of the science that was operative among this crowd, they were basically saying, without realizing it, that causation could be established *"homodemiologically."* The presumptions of heterosexist and political epidemiology would trump the traditional rules of evidence. And those rules could basically be summed up as "Heads I win and tails you lose." "You" basically being gays and eventually blacks.

Lauritsen caught the powerful HIV advocates in the act of doublespeak that is common to abnormal, totalitarian science: "Actually, the HIV advocates talked out of both sides of their mouths with regard to Koch's postulates. On the one hand, they disparaged them as in need of 'modification' (read abandonment); on the other hand, they were doing their best to come up with data that would satisfy at least the first postulate." (*PBP* p.145)

Duesberg's opponents at the forum included a living, breathing example of scientific conflict of interest, William Haseltine, a scientist who was in the process of making a lot of money from HIV testing, and Anthony Fauci, the empire-building Director of NIAID.

At the amfAR Forum, Fauci and others played a curious unfair game with Duesberg. Hypocritically they accused Duesberg of citing research that was out of date even though it was basically *the same research quoted at that time* by the AIDS establishment. On the other hand, when Duesberg would ask Fauci and others for actual references to support *their* statements at the amfAR forum, he was "rudely rebuffed," and according to Lauritsen, they tried to shore up their viewpoint about HIV with unpublished data, or "their own private facts." (*PBP* p.147) "Private facts" not on the public record are another sure sign that AIDS was a manifestation of the opposite world of abnormal, totalitarian and sociopathic science. Unfortunately, their private facts about AIDS were also connected to each other by a private scientific logic.

The 800-pound gorilla at the amfAR forum was the fact that evidence of HIV could *not be found in all AIDS patients*, which should have been strong—damning even—evidence that HIV couldn't possibly be the cause of AIDS, that is, if Kuhnian normal science was being practiced. As scientist Marcel Beluda pointed out at the meeting, "sometimes even a single exception is sufficient to disprove a theory." . . . This is the crux of the matter. The virus cannot be found in all cases of AIDS." (*PBP* p.151) One could say that still believing that HIV is the cause of AIDS in the face of evidence that it could not be found in all patients is Exhibit A that delusion and denial were running the show.

Fauci's answer belongs in a beginner's textbook on the card tricks of abnormal science: "Fauci responded to Beluda by saying that a good lab was able to isolate the virus in 90-100% of the cases, that there was 'no question about it.' Fauci did not provide a reference to published data, nor did he indicate what the 'good labs' were, or how exactly they differed from the not-so-good labs." (*PBP* p.151) References belong to the abandoned Kuhnian world of normal science.

Duesberg made a number of arguments, based on his years as one of the celebrated deans of retroviral research, about why HIV could not possibly be the cause of AIDS.

Lauritsen wrote that Fauci's presentation "while aspiring to be a point-by-point rebuttal to Duesberg, consisted mainly of disconnected assertions, delivered in a tone of petulant indignation. Epidemiological studies conducted in San Francisco and unpublished laboratory reports seemed to be the basis of most of his statements. So far as I could tell, he understood none of Duesberg's arguments . . . ." (*PBP* p.155)

The role of the AIDS politics of epidemiology in AIDS research showed itself dramatically at the forum. According to Lauritsen, "In the question period, Beluda asked if the evidence were sufficient that HIV is necessary for the development of AIDS, Fauci replied that he hoped the epidemiologists would answer that question." (*PBP* p.157) (Given the political and heterosexist nature of AIDS epidemiology, one could guess how *that* was going to turn out.)

The most shocking and downright hilarious episode at the forum occurred when Harvard Medical School's William Haseltine spoke. Lauritsen reported that "His presentation was devoted largely to personal attacks on Duesberg." (*PBP* p.157) Ironically, *he* accused Duesberg of resorting to personal attacks. In another telltale moment of abnormal and totalitarian science, Lauritsen caught Haseltine trying to explain away the anomalies about the evidence of AIDS in men and women in America: "He attacked Duesberg's 'paradox,' that the AIDS virus seemed to be able to discriminate between boys and girls, by saying that this was not true outside the U.S.—in Africa, about equal numbers of men and women develop AIDS. (He seemed oblivious to the paradox that a microbe should be able to discriminate in one country, but not in another.)" (*PBP* p.158) In a memorable moment that perfectly captured the essence of the past and future of AIDS research, Haseltine showed the audience a slide of a graph that was meant to absolutely demolish Duesberg's argument. The slide was supposed to show a correlation between the rise in HIV titers with the decline of T cells in the progression of AIDS. There was just one small problem: Duesberg quickly noticed that *there were no units on the vertical axis of the slide.* Haseltine was angry and flustered by the charge and had to ask Dr. Robert Redfield, an AIDS researcher from the military, how the slide was prepared. At the forum Redfield said, "different measurements were used," but later that night at a post-forum party, according to Lauritsen's report, Redfield told Duesberg and other people at the gathering that "the graph had been prepared to illustrate a theoretical possibility. It had no units on it for the simple reason that *it was not based on any data at all*. In other words, the slide was a fake." (*PBP* p.161) That's the kind of ideology-based data that was used to back up the HIV theory of AIDS which changed the course of millions of lives and fostered the HHV-6 catastrophe.

In terms of the habitual use of political epidemiology (or "homo-demiology") rather than real science to deal with AIDS during "Holocaust II," the most disturbing talk was given by Warren Winkelstein, Professor of Biomedical Environmental Health Sciences at U.C. Berkeley. Essentially, he too suggested that AIDS would require *a new kind of science*. According to Lauritsen, "the point of Winkelstein's presentation is that Koch's postulates should be superseded by new standards for establishing the causal relationship between microbes and disease, and that these standards should be based upon 'epidemiology' or, as it were, correlations of various kinds." (*PBP* p.162) If this crowd had superseded traditional science any more than they did, we all would probably be dead. (But wait. There is still time.)

Most of the scientific world was not aware of the degree to which this zany cast of characters was improvising a questionable newfangled science as they went along. And it was being done in a Fauci-style of "petulant indignation," to reprise Lauritsen's very apt phrase. That it was all dependent on a loosey-goosey, all too subjective political "discipline" like epidemiology should have disturbed Lauritsen's sixteen journalistic colleagues who were at the amfAR affair. But there was already a tragically cozy relationship between the media and the abnormal, totalitarian and sociopathic scientists of "Holocaust II." For three decades as the HIV/AIDS paradigm held sway, most of the reporters who covered AIDS were a self-satisfied, inattentive, group-thinking, intellectually slothful bunch who wouldn't know independent, journalistic due diligence if it bit them. A corrupt scientific community could totally depend on them.

Lauritsen's eyewitness record of the forum (originally published in *New York Native*) was an important contribution to the history of the flakey beginnings of the science and totalitarian politics of AIDS. His diligent and critical reporting is proof that *not every journalist* was hoodwinked by these charlatans. He didn't buy into this new improvised epidemiological science that the AIDS establishment was dumping on the public: "I do not accept the proposition that Koch's postulates should be abandoned in favor of epidemiological correlations. This would be a step backward, a step away from scientific rigor, a step towards impressionism and confusion." (*PBP* p.162) Lauritsen didn't acknowledge it, but it was also a big heterosexist (and ultimately racist) step backwards.

Like many others, Lauritsen came face to face with totalitarian, abnormal, and sociopathic science. Unfortunately, even though he was openly gay himself, he didn't grasp the manner in which the infernal game was being played—or what the game was actually concealing. He didn't fully perceive the homodemiological underpinnings of what was happening before his very eyes. But he definitely grasped the fact that the science of the budding AIDS Establishment was utterly bogus. He concluded his report by writing "I am more convinced than ever that HIV is not the cause of AIDS. If the HIV advocates were sure of their hypothesis, they would want to enlighten Duesberg and the rest of us; they would want to publish their arguments in a proper scientific journal complete with references. They would not need to resort to stonewalling, deception, and personal abuse." (*PBP* p.168) Science had been supplanted by totalitarian petulance.

The 1988 amfAR Forum was another one of the tragic "What if?" moments in the dark history of AIDS. What if the reporters had looked closer at Haseltine's fake slide and realized that it was the tip of the iceberg, a little like the scientific version of the Watergate break-in that would have led them to a much bigger crime if they only followed the lies? What if they had reported that AIDS science, as practiced by Anthony Fauci, was simply out-to-lunch? What if they had been independent enough to notice that epidemiology was overplaying its arrogant, biased hand and that, in reality, it is actually a soft, subjective enterprise vulnerable to political manipulation? Why was it beyond the pale to wonder if this defensive and cranky gathering was actually the expression of some rather unsavory feelings and hostilities directed at the so-called beneficiaries of this new kind of "science," namely the gay community? Maybe someone should have asked if there was something funky about a group of hostile, arrogant, white heterosexual mostly-male scientists performing their jerry-built kind of seat-of-the-pants epidemiological science on gays. Wasn't that a formula for all kinds of prurient, heterosexist pseudoscientific mischief if ever there was one? In terms of majorities doing their science on minorities, hadn't anyone ever heard of Nazi science or the Tuskegee Syphilis Experiment? God only knows what personal sexual issues were being acted out by this elite motley crew under the cover of what has turned out to be highfalutin retroviral claptrap. Why didn't anyone other than Lauritsen notice the peculiar, unscientific defensiveness of the whole affair, i.e. that the ladies had protested too much? And most importantly for the main event, why was HHV-6, which had been discovered in AIDS patients two years before that curious amfAR forum, not put on the table for discussion?

Fauci believed in the kind of transparency and communications with the public that are typical of abnormal science. He laid out the draconian media policy that he would maintain for the nearly thirty years he ran the totalitarian HIV/AIDS empire in a brief piece he wrote for the AAAS Observer on September 1, 1989.

Fauci wrote, "When I first got involved in AIDS research, I was reluctant to deal with the press. I thought it was not dignified. But there was a lot of distortion by those who were speaking to the press so I changed my mind." The "distortion" was, of course, coming from those who didn't agree with the very dignified Fauci about the etiology of AIDS. Fauci had his own idea of what the media's responsibility is. He notes that his interpretation of what the media is supposed to do "doesn't even jibe with what competent journalists think." He asserts that the big dilemma for journalists is between what is "important" and what is "newsworthy" and he notes that they sometimes "are not the same." He whines about the fact that journalists are more interested in the latest story of a cure than the "magnificent science" involving the regulatory genes of HIV.

Fauci describes what he thinks is the hierarchy of media. It ranges from *The New York Times* and *The Washington Post* all the way down to publications that "care only about sales or have axes to grind." (He had yet to face the unwashed barbarians of the blogs and the commenters of the online forums.) One can safely assume that the publications with axes to grind were the ones who didn't agree with the axe that the petulant Fauci himself was grinding.

It is amusing that Fauci pontificated in 1989 that "the media are no place for amateurs, particularly when talking about a public health problem of the magnitude of AIDS." Especially when one considers the magnitude of the HHV-6 public health problem that this very self-reverential scientist (that Bruce Nussbaum described as "lackluster") himself helped create for the whole human race. While Fauci would make one think that the real problem in AIDS journalism was the clownish journalist who can't spell "retrovirus" or one who didn't listen carefully after asking questions, his real quarry in this peevish little piece is something far more serious. Fauci's real problem was journalists who not only *could* spell "retrovirus" but could also actually hear what he was saying *all too well*. The kind of journalists who also knew things about retroviruses and listened to what he was saying so closely and critically that they could make life unpleasant for Fauci and his powerful AIDS cronies by asking inconvenient questions.

Fauci's nose should have grown several feet when he wrote, "We know that reporters must consult more than a single source and make room for dissenting opinions." What was yet to come in the AAAS piece made that one of the biggest fibs in the history of American science. Under the pretense of giving us a little lesson in the relationship between science and the media and warning that people too often believe what they read in the papers, Fauci reveals his real agenda: "One striking example is Peter Duesberg's theory that HIV is not the cause of AIDS. I laughed at that for a while, but it led to a lot of public concern that HIV was a hoax. The theory had a great deal of credibility just on the basis of news coverage." This was Fauci being intellectually dishonest on a couple of counts. Duesberg never said it was a *hoax*. He said it was a *mistake*. A hoax is a whole other ball of wax, and it is an example of using language politically to deliberately misrepresent the opposition. Duesberg wasn't saying something similar to those who say that the landing on the moon was just staged with props and a camera. He was a Nobel-caliber expert on retroviruses pointing out the deficiencies of the HIV theory of AIDS using basic logic and analyzing the available evidence. And blaming the media for the credibility given to Duesberg's ideas ignored all the scientists, (eventually including two Nobel Prize winners), who publicly supported Duesberg's skepticism. Fauci was Trumpian in that he was essentially accusing those who spotted his fake science as being purveyors of fake news.

Fauci then introduces us to the smarter member of his family, his sister: "My barometer of what the general public is thinking is my sister Denise. My sister Denise is an intelligent woman who reads avidly, listens to the radio, and watches television, but she is not a scientist. When she calls me and questions my integrity as a scientist, there really is a problem. Denise has called me at least ten times about Peter Duesberg. She says, 'Anthony'—she is the only one who calls me Anthony, 'are you sure he's wrong?' That's the power of putting someone on television or in the press, although there is virtually nothing in his argument that makes any scientific sense." This captures how touchy Fauci was. No one was questioning his "integrity as a scientist." His sister was simply asking him if it was *possible* that he was wrong, and the answer that would have shown some scientific integrity would have been, "Yes, my dear Denise, it is always possible that I'm wrong, although I think the evidence suggests I'm right." The fact that Fauci took this *soooooo* personally speaks volumes about the petulant chip-on-the-shoulder attitude problems of those in charge of AIDS. Fauci put it all on the line. Questioning his so-called science was a threat to his very being. It shouldn't surprise anyone that he was willing to viciously fight for so long during "Holocaust II" to keep everyone from seeing what a house of cards he had helped build. The funny thing is that in a number of ways this scientific masterpiece suggests he *did* have serious problems in the integrity department. (Between the lines of the piece Freudian historians may one day even find the glimmer of a guilty conscience.)

Fauci, like most of the crowd that gave us "Holocaust II," knew only too well what normal, nontotalitarian science is supposed to look like: "People are especially confused when they see divergent viewpoints about the same thing. They do not understand that the beauty of science is that it is self-corroborating and self-correcting, that it is important for scientists to be wrong." (If that's really the case, Fauci *was* indeed doing something incredibly important with

HIV.) It was actually Fauci who didn't understand that the whole process of self-corroboration and self-correction was being short-circuited by the totalitarian hijinks of the touchy HIV/AIDS establishment that was growing more dominant by the day. The very tone of Fauci's piece, its extraordinary imperiousness and presumptuousness about the stupidity of the public, points to the fundamental problem for a society in which arrogant and dishonest elite scientific communities have more and more power. Fauci would not only be the judge and jury of what was true in science, but he also wanted to decide *who* deserved to write about it and *what* they should write. He clearly left no room for the possibility that the really good journalists would be the kind that questioned what *he* had to say.

Fauci also made it pretty clear in the piece that, try as they might, AIDS critics and dissidents would get absolutely nowhere because he was permanently stacking the deck against them: "The lack of clear-cut black-or-white answers plagues the biomedical sciences compared with the physical sciences. Stanley Pons and Martin Fleishmann said they had achieved nuclear fusion at room temperature. Other scientists tried, but they could not reproduce it. Bingo it's over. But because we cannot ethically do clinical trials to establish that he is wrong, I am probably going to be answering Peter Duesberg for the rest of my life." Someone near him should have tried to convince Fauci that it wasn't all about *him*. One also loves the presumption that he was going to control the official etiology of AIDS *for the rest of his life*. Unfortunately, *he almost has*. Beyond the breathtaking megalomania of the statement is the stupidity that the only way to show HIV wasn't the cause of AIDS was to do clinical trials with patients. All it would have taken would have been a few patients with AIDS *who had no evidence of HIV*. The only people that would be hurt by the implications of that finding would be the dishonest and incompetent scientists, like Fauci, whose undeserved reputations and incomes had depended upon the HIV theory. Those HIV-negative patients would be forthcoming—in spades. In fact those patients were basically the very immune-compromised Chronic Fatigue Syndrome patients a doctor named Richard DuBois had seen in his Atlanta practice *before* the socio-epidemiological construction of the heterosexist and racist HIV/AIDS paradigm.

Hillary Johnson reported on the DuBois Atlanta cases in *Osler's Web: Inside the Labyrinth of Chronic Fatigue Syndrome Epidemic*, her epic work of journalism detailing the CDC's failure to acknowledge the true nature of the Chronic Fatigue Syndrome epidemic. It is now all too painfully obvious that the DuBois cases—with the telltale signs of hypergammaglobulinemia, t-cell perturbations and persistent reactivated EBV and CMV infections—were the beginning of the real AIDS/CFS/HHV-6 disaster. According to Johnson, in 1980 Richard DuBois "saw a thirteen-year old girl who suffered from a seemingly endless case of mono. As the months passed, he identified several more cases of the curious syndrome in his practice." (*OW* p.7) He wasn't alone. Johnson reported that he was in touch with other clinicians who had seen similar cases and he and his colleagues eventually had a research article published about it in the Southern Medical Journal in 1984, the same year the big consequential government mistake of certifying HIV as the official AIDS virus occurred. According to Johnson, "they [DuBois and his colleagues] had believed that they were describing a new syndrome, one that would have increasing importance and was worthy of national attention." (*OW* p.7) The DuBois patients morphed into the millions of Chronic Fatigue Syndrome and HHV-6 patients that Fauci and his organization (which was supposed to handle infectious diseases) were willfully ignoring while building their Potemkin HIV/AIDS empire.

At the end of Fauci's little *AAAS* piece comes the shot across the media's bow from the tiny AIDS czar: "Scientists need to get more sophisticated about expressing themselves. But the media have to do their homework. They have got to learn the issues and the background. And they should realize that their accuracy is noted by the scientific community. Journalists who make too many mistakes, who are sloppy, are going to find that their access to scientists may diminish." In other words, the scientists that journalists reported on were going to be the high-handed and underhanded final arbiters of what the public knows about science. They could decide to cut off journalists *they* defined as making mistakes and being sloppy, and one would assume that one of those sloppy mistakes would probably entail giving any coverage to scientists like Peter Duesberg, who raised serious questions about what was being called good science by

Fauci and the rest of the HIV/AIDS establishment. Fauci was basically saying that he and his cronies would only be accountable to themselves which is the hermetically-sealed, closed-community essence of what should be called totalitarian, abnormal, and ultimately sociopathic science.

If anyone ever makes a serious film about "Holocaust II" it will have to include the shocking revelation (already referred to above) that came to light during the Eighth International Conference on AIDS in Amsterdam during July of 1992. Its historic importance rivals that of the Wannsee conference during World War II or the Gulf of Tonkin incident. It was *the moment of no turning back*, the moment a fateful line was crossed, a life of virtual pseudoscientific crime against humanity was virtually signed onto and those responsible for "Holocaust II" lost all forms of plausible deniability. AIDS almost overnight became AIDSgate and a very unique Nazi-like biomedical and epidemiological assault against humanity. And, ultimately, the man who stood at the center of the developments that came out of Amsterdam was Anthony Fauci. Before Amsterdam one might be able to say that Fauci wasn't exactly the Bernie Madoff of the biomedical Ponzi Scheme that maintained AIDS, Chronic Fatigue Syndrome and the HHV-6 spectrum catastrophe. *But not after Amsterdam.*

Hillary Johnson provided a detailed account of what happened at that Amsterdam conference in her book. She recounts how the conference was electrified by news from a small press conference that was held in California at which a scientist named "Subhir Gupta, a University of California immunologist, reported he had isolated particles of a previously unknown retrovirus from an HIV-negative, ailing sixty-six-year-old woman, her symptomless daughter and six other patients." (*OW* p.600) According to Johnson, "Investigators and the lay press gathered in Holland were riveted by Gupta's announcement that the older woman suffered from an 'AIDS-like' condition wherein a component of her immune system, a subset of T-cells called CD4 cells, were severely depleted. In addition, she had suffered a bout of *Pneumocystis carinii* pneumonia, a so-called opportunistic infection that afflicted many AIDS patients whose CD4 cells were depleted." (*OW* p.600)

That announcement was soon outdone by a flurry of shocking revelations from additional scientists at the Amsterdam conference who had "findings of retrovirus particles in HIV-negative patients with AIDS-like symptoms." (*OW* p.601) A near panic was almost set off internationally by the possibility that there was a second previously unrecognized AIDS epidemic on the horizon that was caused by a non-HIV agent. (*OW* p.601)

According to Johnson, it turned out that the Centers for Disease Control *was already aware* of such HIV-negative cases of an AIDS-like illness. (*OW* p.601) Johnson reported that months before Gupta's press conference two CDC scientists had reported on "six cases of non-HIV positive AIDS." (*OW* p.601) Their conclusion was that "HIV may not be the only infectious cause of immune deficiency." (*OW* p.601) Two AIDS viruses? A gay one and a straight one? OMG!

The HIV-negative cases of AIDS-like illness set off an explosion in the press, most notably from Lawrence Altman, the reporter who guided *The New York Times* dreadful, sycophantic reporting on AIDS throughout "Holocaust II." In the *Times* Altman wrote that the CDC's embarrassment was "huge because the agency had lost control over the dissemination of new information in the field of AIDS." (*OW* p.602) (That anyone at the *Times* could stress the importance of a government agency *controlling information* with a straight face is pretty amazing and revealing.)

According to Johnson, the CFS research community was especially fascinated by the fact that the Gupta HIV-negative AIDS-like cases were Chronic Fatigue Syndrome sufferers. (*OW* p.604) And for anyone following the bizarre scientific politics of AIDS, it was interesting that Gupta's colleague, the man who supposedly isolated the new retrovirus was none other than Zaki Salahuddin, the scientist who had worked for Robert Gallo and had faced criminal charges for creating a company that garnered illegal self-dealt income from his position at the National Cancer Institute. Johnson reported that when Salahuddin was asked whether HIV-negative AIDS might be Chronic Fatigue Syndrome, he said, "It's a fair statement. But I'm not a prophet. Time and money [are] required for this." (*OW* p.604) Johnson also reported, "Salahuddin confirmed that he and Gupta, who had a cohort of CFS patients in his clinical practice and who had presented papers on the immunology of CFS at medical conferences on the disease, had discussed the possibility that CFS and non-HIV positive AIDS were the same disease." (*OW* p.604) Also, according to Johnson, the non-HIV positive AIDS cases caught the attention of Paul Cheney, one of the two pioneering Lake Tahoe Chronic Fatigue Syndrome researchers. Johnson wrote, "For years he had observed that some CFS patients met the government's defining criteria for AIDS on every count except infection with human immunodeficiency virus." (*OW* p.604) He also told Johnson that "It was hardly unheard of . . . to diagnose the kinds of opportunistic infections that torment AIDS victims—maladies like thrush, candida and pneumonia—in CFS." (*OW* p.604) In the world of normal science this would have been called "the smoking gun."

The AIDS conference in 1992 should have been one of those great moments in normal science as described by Thomas Kuhn. It could have been a moment when disturbing "anomalies" should have attracted the "attention of a scientific community." (*The Structure of Scientific Revolutions* p.ix) But this would not be a moment for AIDS research that "the profession can no longer evade anomalies that subvert the existing tradition of scientific practice" which would "begin the extraordinary investigations that lead the profession at last to a new set of commitments, a new basis for the practice of science." (*SSR* p.6) This would *not* be one of those eureka moments in science characterized by "the community's rejection of one time-honored scientific theory in favor of another incompatible with it." (*SSR* p.6) There would be no "transformation of the world within which science was done." (*SSR* p.6) There would be no "change in the rules governing the prior practice." (*SSR* p.7) As a result of what happened in Amsterdam, scientists would *not* alter their "conception of entities with which [they] had long been familiar." (*SSR* p.7) Amsterdam would *not* cause the AIDS researchers' worlds to be "qualitatively transformed as well as quantitatively enriched by fundamental novelties of either fact or theory." (*SSR* p.7) After the revelations of HIV-negative AIDS cases, the researchers would still *not* give up their "shared paradigm." (*SSR* p.11) No new AIDS (or Chronic Fatigue Syndrome = AIDS) paradigm was allowed to reveal itself in Amsterdam and subsequently be fairly examined and debated. The HIV-negative cases of AIDS would *not* be recognized as an important scientific surprise that would lead scientists "to see nature in a different way." (*SSR* p.53) The scientific world of AIDS researchers did not change "in an instant" (*SSR* p.56) the way it might have if AIDS research was taking place in the world of normal science. (And consequently, immune-system-destroying HHV-6 would remain locked in the basement of "science.")

Tragically, the HIV-negative AIDS cases were not a wake-up call for the scientists that "something had gone wrong" and hence the anomalous cases were not "a prelude to discovery." (*SSR* p.57) Even though the HIV-negative AIDS cases "violated deeply entrenched expectations," (*SSR* p.59) they were not allowed to change *anything* about the AIDS paradigm. In Kuhn's world of normal science, the "traditional pursuit prepares the way for its own change." (*SSR* p.65) Amsterdam showed that AIDS research was being conducted in normal science's cockamamie opposite world, one that should be called "abnormal, totalitarian and sociopathic science." Even if the HIV-negative AIDS cases could have ultimately led to a new paradigm that was "able to account for wider range of natural phenomena," (*SSR* p.66) they were dead on arrival. No "novel theory" about AIDS which was a "direct response to crisis" (*SSR* p.75) was allowed to emerge because the abnormal, totalitarian, and sociopathic science of AIDS was *politically invulnerable* to crisis. At that historic conference there was never any chance that the HIV/AIDS theory would be "declared invalid" even though a new "CFS is a form of AIDS" paradigm was staring out at the conference from the new anomalous data and was a perfectly credible "alternate candidate." (*SSR* p.77) Kuhn wrote that the decision to reject one paradigm is always simultaneously the decision to accept another, and the judgment leading to that decision involves the comparison of both paradigms with nature and with each other." (*SSR* p.77) The HIV-negative AIDS cases were *not allowed* to catalyze that kind of fertile intellectual process in Amsterdam. Kuhn would probably argue that absent a new paradigm to examine and accept in Amsterdam, there was no exit from the HIV/AIDS paradigm because "To reject one paradigm without simultaneously substituting another is to reject science itself." (*SSR* p.79) In a way, much of what happened at the

AIDS conference was based on appeals to something quite characteristic of the AIDS establishment and abnormal science: *authority*. The petulant HIV/AIDS authorities basically said, "Nothing here, folks. Please move along." And unfortunately, the scientific community and the media (with a few notable exceptions) did exactly that. Kuhnian *anomaly* didn't turn into Kuhnian *crisis* and that in turn did not explode into Kuhnian *scientific revolution* as it should have. The HIV-negative cases in Amsterdam should have led to a period of what Kuhn called "extraordinary science" (*SSR* p.82) in which "the rules of normal science become increasingly blurred." (*SSR* p.83) (Although one could argue that the rules of AIDS research already actually were a shocking chocolate mess.) Amsterdam would not be the transformative moment when "formerly standard solutions of solved problems are called into question." (*SSR* p.83) The conference should have been a fruitful time when scientists were "terribly confused." (*SSR* p.84) If things had gone the way they should have at that conference, the assembled AIDS researchers would have ultimately changed their view of "the field, its methods, and its goals." (*SSR* p.85) HHV-6 might have been allowed to reveal itself in all its pathological glory. And the scientists who had given us the HIV paradigm would have been revealed in all their vainglory.

Had the science of Amsterdam been *normal*, both AIDS research and Chronic Fatigue Syndrome research might have morphed into one unified discipline. The dismantling of the "Chronic Fatigue Syndrome isn't AIDS" paradigm should have begun in earnest. HHV-6 (and its spectrum or family) might have emerged quickly as the unifying viral agent(s) of those two epidemics which should have always been considered one in the first place. And those two epidemics were just the tip of the HHV-6 iceberg. What happened in Amsterdam was a virtual nosological and epidemiological crime. It was the deliberate attempt to use *sheer political force* to make a legitimate scientific crisis disappear. As a result, scientists would not turn to what Kuhn describes as a "philosophical analysis as a device for unlocking the riddles of their field." (*SSR* p.88) "Philosophical analysis" was Greek to this confederacy of dunces. The crisis was not allowed to play itself out and would not loosen what Kuhn calls the "stereotypes" and provide "the incremental data necessary for a fundamental paradigm shift." (*SSR* p.89) There would be no Kuhnian "transition from normal to extraordinary research." (*SSR* p.91) It should have been painfully clear in Amsterdam "that an existing paradigm [had] ceased to function adequately in the exploration of an aspect of nature to which that paradigm itself had previously led the way." (*SSR* p.92)

A potentially life-saving scientific revolution in AIDS and CFS research was politically nipped in the bud in Amsterdam and in the months that followed. No "new theory" was allowed to surface that would "permit predictions that are different from those derived from its predecessor" (*SSR* p.97) Kuhn asserted that "the price of significant scientific advance is a commitment that runs the risk of being wrong."(*SSR* p.101) Those in control of the abnormal science of AIDS had no interest in engaging in *any* kind of science that would prove *them* wrong. "Wrong" was not in their cultish vocabulary. They had bet their white heterosexual male professional reputations and the credibility of American science on their ridiculous and dangerous HIV/AIDS and "Chronic Fatigue Syndrome is not AIDS" paradigms. Fake dividends of their scientific Ponzi Scheme would be paid out for decades.

What happened in Amsterdam was the opening and almost simultaneously closing of a Pandora's Box of incredibly important scientific questions and implications. The person most responsible for keeping that box closed then and for the next two decades was the de facto AIDS Czar, the tantrum-prone Anthony Fauci. This may have been the last chance for Fauci and the HIV/AIDS establishment to turn back from the precipice of the HHV-6 spectrum catastrophe. But even his sister Denise could not save him from securing this dark place in history.

According to Hillary Johnson, "On August 15, federal scientists convened a meeting in Atlanta to discuss the emerging health threat of non-HIV positive AIDS. In the three weeks since Sudhir Gupta's paper on his isolation of a new intracisternal retrovirus in a handful of cases, the number of reported cases had risen from approximately thirty to fifty. Nobel prize winners, members of the National Academy of Sciences, CDC's AIDS administrators, and Anthony Fauci, head of the National Institute of Allergy and Infectious

Diseases, formed a panel to query scientists Gupta, David Ho of the Aaron Diamond AIDS Center in New York and Jeffrey Laurence, a Cornell Medical College cancer and AIDS specialist and associate professor of medicine, each of whom had been studying cases of the syndrome and discovered evidence of retroviral infection in patients." (*OW* p.606) It didn't matter how many brilliant scientists from different institutions were queried at the meeting, because their mindsets about HIV were all the same. It was like a mini-Woodstock of groupthink. There was no turning back from the HIV/AIDS and "Chronic Fatigue Syndrome *is not* AIDS" paradigm. The carved-in-stone paradigm was eight years old at that point and the nation's heterosexist and racist AIDS propaganda and public health policies had been built on its assumptions. The gay and black communities had been herded into it like cattle into a train. It was another moment in abnormal science in which the privileged and paranoid foxes had formed a panel to investigate the henhouse.

The manner in which Fauci and his colleagues basically covered up the shocking anomalies of HIV-negative AIDS was relatively simple and Orwellian: as previously noted, they disingenuously gave the HIV-negative cases an obfuscatory new name (Idiopathic CD4 T lymphocytopenia or ICL) and they insisted by fiat that they were not really AIDS cases. The HIV/AIDS elite insisted that because there was no unifying geographic or chronological "risk factor" (OW P.603) to be found in these ordinary Americans and they shared no official AIDS risk factors, there was no HIV-negative AIDS or AIDS-like epidemic covertly occurring in the general population. Fauci's concerned sister Denise would not have to lose sleep at night.

Because the "Chronic Fatigue Syndrome *is not* AIDS" paradigm was not challenged by what happened at the Amsterdam Conference in 1992, for at least another two more decades, the Chronic Fatigue Syndrome patients were locked into their pathetic heterosexist wild goose chase to find a cause while constantly avoiding the obvious links between their medical issues and AIDS. They had Tony Fauci's blessing for that fool's errand. His basic attitude toward CFS was that people shouldn't be ashamed of being told that their problem was psychiatric, (*OW* p.334) which was how the disease was deceptively framed by the government for nearly three decades. And of course, they were just the canaries in the HHV-6 mine. Everyone suffering from multi-systemic problems of the HHV-6 spectrum (like multiple sclerosis, fibromyalgia, autism, and even Morgellons) would ultimately pay a heavy price for the intellectual dishonesty and legerdemain of the 1992 AIDS conference.

Fauci and his colleagues told the public that the HIV-negative cases of AIDS-like illness were rare, but of course it all depended on disease definitions and *who* was doing the defining and counting. Fauci disingenuously sent out a call that summer asking that all HIV-negative cases be reported immediately *to him*. An editorial in *New York Native* heeded his call: "Last week Anthony Fauci of the National Institute of Allergy and Infectious Diseases asked that all cases of HIV-negative AIDS be reported to him. We reported thirteen million American cases. That's the estimate of the number of cases of Chronic Fatigue and Immune Dysfunction, a condition that research (if anyone bothers to read it) suggests is essentially HIV-negative AIDS." (*OW* p.605)

The editorial had no impact on Anthony Fauci and it would not be the only time he would ignore the *New York Native* during "Holocaust II."

One could ultimately say that Denise Fauci's petulant brother himself represented one of the most significant scientific paradigm shifts, one that moved the whole world from normal to abnormal, totalitarian, and sociopathic science. During the Fauci years, The Age of Scientific Racketeering began in earnest. Bernie Madoff has a twin in science whose Ponzi Scheme is a gift that keeps on giving.

Afterword to the Fauci Chapter

Scientific totalitarianism is the background music of Anthony Fauci's brilliant and long-lasting Ponzi scheme. A so-called liberal democracy like America demands a covert form of scientific totalitarianism that does not scare the horses of oversight and public opinion. Fauci knew how to manipulate the levers of institutional power and image-making in ways that Bernie Madoff would envy. For a scientific Ponzi scheme to prevail in America and Europe, nobody must recognize that they have acquiesced to a major medical and scientific fraud. Doctors must follow protocols established by the HIV/AIDS Ponzi scheme and patients must not question them. Sanctions should stand at the ready if they do. Nobody must see the telltale signs of fraud, deceit, and censorship. Fauci knew the tricks required to turn ivy-league-educated elite journalists into servile puppets and perky stenographers. I coined the term "Bob Club" to describe the sycophantic journalists who enabled the massive scientific fraud of disgraced National Cancer Institute researcher Robert Gallo. The "Tony Club" is even worse and consequential in ways that will take medical historians generations to fully illuminate. A long list of servile journalists who were chummy with Fauci and enabled his Ponzi scheme will have a lot to answer for. An intimidating voice, a good haircut, and suits that fit well go a long way in science especially if you are as skilled in the art of veiled and not-so-veiled threats as Fauci is.

Laziness is not a Fauci flaw. It took a great deal of industriousness to cover up the role of the HHV-6/7/8 family of viruses in "AIDS," Chronic Fatigue Syndrome and a myriad of immune disorders that constitute the real "AIDS" epidemic that the Ponzi scheme conceals from the public. To keep the entire NIH establishment from dealing with Chronic Fatigue Syndrome and its relationship to AIDS for almost four decades took a great deal of persistent effort.

Fauci is not stupid. There is no way that some part of him didn't recognize that serious Chronic Fatigue Syndrome research would have easily brought down his whole HIV house of cards if it had been officially acknowledged. Even noting publicly that it was uncanny the way any little bit of Chronic Fatigue Syndrome research (and there is tons of it) showed the illness was similar to AIDS would have threatened the Fauci Ponzi scheme. The HIV house of cards and the wall that separates AIDS and Chronic Fatigue Syndrome are the Fauci legacy. The recognition that he got AIDS wrong because he got Chronic Fatigue Syndrome wrong and vice versa would have turned him into an instant disgrace in the eyes of his family and friends. The egregious self-esteem he had carefully nurtured from his early days in Brooklyn would be a plate of Bethesda toast.

In my career as the publisher of *New York Native* (1980-1997), I had one phone conversation with Anthony Fauci in which I heard his petulance and thin-skinned nature in real time. I called him after I had written an editorial that was critical of Fauci in the form of a satirical poem. As readers probably already suspect, Dr. Fauci does not have much of a sense of humor. Especially when it is directed at him by someone in the media who does not know their place. I suspect that his desk at the National Institutes of Allergy and Infectious Diseases is surrounded by eggshells. I believe that even though my newspaper went out of business in 1997, *New York Native* remains a thorn in his psyche to this very day. I doubt that he can hear the words "Chronic Fatigue Syndrome," "HHV-6," or "Peter Duesberg" without thinking of *New York Native.*

Two of my reporters paid a price for their association with *New York Native.* He was dramatically rude to one reporter when she showed up on the same TV show with him. He refused to shake the hand of another reporter when he was introduced to him at a medical conference. Not surprising since I have already pointed out in the chapter above that Fauci basically said that members of the media would lose precious access if they didn't play ball.

I will give credit to Fauci for being astute in recognizing my newspaper as his bête noire because it does contain all the journalistic ingredients necessary for his eventual downfall. In my book about *New York Native, The Chronic Fatigue Syndrome Epidemic Cover-up*, you can watch the evolution of the Fauci Ponzi scheme from the beginning of the AIDS epidemic into the early years of the deftly handled Chronic Fatigue Syndrome cover-up.

From my experience covering the CDC and Fauci's antics I now believe that scientific totalitarianism is fertile ground for medical and scientific Ponzi schemes. And when you find scientific Ponzi schemes, you know you have also encountered a culture of scientific totalitarianism. From watching Fauci and his public health puppets closely, I have constructed a list of the elements necessary for a successful public health Ponzi scheme.

1. Nosological fraud. (That's the branch of medicine dealing with the classification of disease. It is ground zero for public health fraud.)

2. Epidemiological fraud.

3. Virological fraud.

4. Treatment fraud. (Treatments that harm more than they heal or conceal more than they reveal.)

5. Public health policy fraud.

6. Concealment of negative scientific data and paradigm-challenging anomalies.

7. Use of an elite network of "old boys" and pseudo-activist provocateurs to censor critics and whistleblowers.

8. Chronic obscurantism.

9. If necessary, vigilantism and witch-hunts against any intellectuals, scientists, or citizens who constitute any form of resistance to the Ponzi scheme.

10. A subservient scientific press that is used as a conveyor belt for the Ponzi scheme's propaganda.

While you could say that it took a village to put these elements into place, there really is only one person who has been able to control all the aspects of the Ponzi scheme the way Leonard Bernstein controlled an orchestra. Anthony Fauci has been richly rewarded for his ability to keep this Ponzi scheme going, just as Bernie Madoff was for his. These are just some of the awards Fauci received:

1979: Arthur S. Flemming Award

1990: International Chiron Award for Biomedical Research and Training, from Accademia Nazionale di Medicina - Italy

1995: Ernst Jung Prize (shared with Samuel A. Wells, Jr.)[9]

2002: Albany Medical Center Prize

2005: National Medal of Science

2005: American Association of Immunologists Lifetime Achievement Award

2007: Mary Woodard Lasker Public Service Award

2008: Presidential Medal of Freedom

2013: Robert Koch Gold Medal

2013: Prince Mahidol Award

Fauci is one of the highest paid people in the government. I leave it to historians to sort out how much he made from his scientific Ponzi scheme. Journalist Terry Michael was working on a book about Fauci's ill-gotten gains but, unfortunately, died before he could finish it.

If you search Google for articles or blogs that are critical of Fauci, except for a few notable examples (my work and Hillary Johnson's) you will come up empty handed. Journalism about Fauci tends to be uninformed, uncritical, and lionizing. The most iconic piece about him was the canonization he received from a nun. In a Catholic News Agency article, Sister Joan L. Roccasalvo wrote, "Dr. Fauci is blessed with a first-class temperament crowning his other achievements. This, despite his own admission of being a perfectionist. Some years ago, at the height of the AIDS controversy, I listened to him delivering a lecture. In the Q&A, one person after the other lashed out at him. Quick to size up, deliberate to respond, this preppy-looking physician answered calmly and without condescension. His style: cool. Later he observed that the audience was lashing out at everyone and not at him in particular. He had walked with them in their pain. He absorbed their pain. Wasn't this Christ's way? And what of St. Luke, the physician, whose gospel is permeated with compassion for the most vulnerable?"

Sister Joan L. Roccasalvo outdid herself when she ended her piece by noting " . . . Dr. Fauci's inspiration cannot be measured. In fact, the beauty of such a life is the surest and most persuasive occasion to form disciples of the Lord and build a better world. God's love shines out from those who, of themselves, are unaware of God's limitless power working in their lives for good. So it is with Anthony Fauci, a man for others, a universal treasure."

To that, one can only say what must be uttered when he speaks at NIH: "Amen." Fauci knew the importance of good public relations.

He could have taught Bernie Madoff a thing or two about working a crowd. If the nuns are on your side you have nothing to worry about. See if you can find a You Tube moment when Rachel Maddow tells Fauci that she thinks he is "a great American."

When Madoff's Ponzi scheme was eventually exposed, it was shocking how obvious the scam was. Boston financial analyst Harry Markopolos, the man who figured out what Madoff was up to, told *60 Minutes*, "It took me five minutes to know that it was a fraud. It took me another almost four hours of mathematical modeling to prove it was a fraud." There was no shortage of people who discerned the glaring irregularities in the "science" that bolstered Fauci's Ponzi scheme. In addition to the reporters at *New York Native*, there was a fascinating group of scientists and intellectuals I discuss in *Peter Duesberg and the Duesbergians*.

In some ways, you could say that Fauci's Ponzi scheme has survived for so long because his critics were too nice. Assuming that norms were being maintained, they were often collegial, hoping that reason would prevail. It would not. It's a shame that Fauci's critics didn't recognize that they were really whistleblowers and scientific crime-fighters. They would politely make their points in a Fauci universe where critics were welcome to get jobs at Starbucks. You can't reason with someone who has Fauci's power and administrative long arms because at all times he is running and protecting a criminal enterprise. His fake science is always covertly fighting for its life.

Two communities especially have failed to grasp the nature of Fauci's HIV Ponzi scheme and paid a terrible price for it: the gay community and the Chronic Fatigue Syndrome community. The gay community and the Chronic Fatigue Syndrome community are now victims of a massive epidemic associated with the HHV-6/7/8 family of viruses. I will have more to say about this in a future book, but anyone who wants to explore the implications of the HHV-6/7/8 epidemic should check out the over 3,000 posts on my website, HHV-6 University.

It's very sad that the Chronic Fatigue Syndrome community has never challenged the HIV/AIDS pseudoscience of Anthony Fauci. While there is a great deal of CFS-related hostility toward Fauci, it generally revolves around *neglect* of Chronic Fatigue Syndrome rather than the *cover-up* of the obvious fact that what has been called AIDS and what has been called Chronic Fatigue Syndrome are really just two different faces of one epidemic driven by the HHV-6/7/8 family of viruses.

When new retroviruses were found in Chronic Fatigue Syndrome patients by scientists Elaine DeFreitas and Judy Mikovits, the work was not discredited just because the retroviruses would show that CFS is real. The truth is that it was undermined because the work threatened to show that Chronic Fatigue Syndrome is just another iteration of the AIDS epidemic. Judy Mikovits, the scientist whose work on XMRV, a mouse retrovirus she claimed to find in CFS patients, was initially the object of international adulation from CFS community. But a scientist connected with the AIDS establishment pulled the rug out from under her work by "de-discovering XMRV," to the great disappointment to CFS patients and activists. If the CFS community knew the truth about AIDS and Fauci's Ponzi scheme, they could have turned the tables on scientists who sent Mikovits into exile because of her retroviral findings. They never asked whether HIV could have been "de-discovered" as the cause of AIDS if it had been as critically vetted as XMRV. I believe that one day historians will conclude that finding a retrovirus in CFS patients would have sent scientists quickly down a slippery slope to an understanding that *HIV is not the real cause of AIDS and AIDS is not HIV disease.* What has been called "AIDS" is on a spectrum of illness caused by the HHV-6/7/8 family of viruses. And that would not be a good development for Anthony Fauci's brilliant Ponzi scheme.

Because Fauci is close to retirement, he may never have to answer for the crisis he has created. I have spent more than half of my life covering his scientific Ponzi scheme. I am hopeful that these books (below) that I have written since the demise of *New York Native* will help future generations clean up the biomedical, political, and cultural mess left by the Fauci Ponzi scheme.

The Chronic Fatigue Syndrome Epidemic Cover-up: How a Little Newspaper Solved the Biggest Scientific and Political Mystery of Our Time

The Chronic Fatigue Syndrome Epidemic Cover-up Volume Two: The Origins of Totalitarianism in Science and Medicine

Peter Duesberg and the Duesbergians: How a Brave and Brilliant Group of Scientists Challenged the AIDS Establishment and Inadvertently Exposed the Chronic Fatigue Syndrome Epidemic

The Closing Argument: A shocking courtroom novella about AIDS, Chronic Fatigue Syndrome, racial injustice and HHV-6, the virus that threatens us all

The Stonewall Massacre

The African Swine Fever Novel

The Black Party: A Dramatic Comedy in Two Acts

The Last Lovers on Earth: Stories from Dark Times

Iron Peter: A Year in the Mythopoetic Life of New York City

Butterfly Ghosts and The New Hippocratic Oath: Earlier and Later Poems

Peter Duesberg

Half a Hero is Better than None

Introduction to the Duesberg Chapter

According to the Holocaust Encyclopedia, "The Nazis believed that male homosexuals were weak, effeminate men who could not fight for the German nation. They saw homosexuals as unlikely to produce children and increase the German birthrate. . . . Because some Nazis believed homo-sexuality was a sickness that could be cured, they designed policies to 'cure' homosexuals of their 'disease' through humiliation and hard work." The Nazis who were "interested in finding a 'cure' for homosexuality" developed a "program to include medical experimentation on homosexual inmates of concentration camps. These experiments caused illness, mutilation and yielded no scientific knowledge."

I refer to what happened to gays during this period as "Holocaust I." According to the United States Holocaust Memorial Museum website, "The severity of the persecution of homosexuals increased after the war's outbreak. In July 1940, Himmler directed that any convicted homosexual who 'seduced more than one partner' be sent to a concentration camp after completing his prison sentence to prevent the homosexual 'contagion' from spreading. After 1942, the SS embarked on an explicit program of 'extermination through work' to destroy Germany's 'habitual criminals.' Some 15,000 prisoners, including homosexuals, were sent from prisons to concentration camps, where nearly all perished within months."

It is also noted on the website that in the camps prisoners were forced to wear "marks of various colors and shapes which allowed guards and camp functionaries to identify them by category. The uniforms of those sentenced as homosexuals bore various identifying marks, including a large black dot" and later a "pink triangle."

The Holocaust Museum also notes, "After the war, homosexual concentration camp prisoners were not acknowledged as victims of Nazi persecutions and reparations were refused."

What I refer to as Holocaust I for gays was a part of what is traditionally referred to as "the Holocaust" or "the Shoah" which was a genocide in which six million Jews were killed. In the Holocaust the homosexuals were not the primary target. Their "crime" was not one of "racial inferiority" but rather for "behavioral inferiority." In Holocaust II they are the primary target.

In his book, *Life Unworthy of Life*, James M. Glass writes about the overlap of the medicalization of the Jews and the gays in Nazi Germany: "It is critical not to underestimate the power of phobia in driving the perception of the Jew as bacillus translated into the public policy of sanitation and infection. Certain stories filtering back to Germany about the condition of the ghettos—the extent of disease, the deadly environment—added to the prevailing view of the Jew as bad blood. A similar attitude prevailed regarding homosexuality. In 1938, Reich Legal Director Hans Frank, who later became head of the General Government in occupied Poland, wrote that homosexuality 'is clearly expressive of a disposition opposed to the normal national community. Homosexual activity means the negation of the community as it must be constituted if the race is not to perish. That is why homosexual behavior in particular, merits no mercy.' In his diary Goebbels called homosexuality a 'cancerous disease.'"

What I call "Holocaust II" is the event that began in 1981, thirty-six years after the German forces surrendered to the Allies: the so-called "AIDS epidemic." As the publisher and editor-in-chief of a gay New York City newspaper called *New York Native,* I was destined to have a front row seat on the tragedy of Holocaust II as it unfolded. In the early years of the epidemic I focused my newspaper continuously on the epidemic and earned nearly universal praise for doing so when most of the media preferred to look the other way. In *Rolling Stone*, David Black said that we deserved a Pulitzer for our early coverage and Randy Shilts also gave it high marks in his bestseller, *And the Band Played On.* I have detailed that coverage and the entire history of my newspaper in my book, *The Chronic Fatigue Syndrome Epidemic Cover-up.*

While my newspaper's early coverage of the epidemic from 1981 to 1983 has been widely celebrated, our commitment to independent investigative and critical reporting about the epidemic eventually earned us the enmity of the government's medical and scientific establishment as well as the AIDS activist community. Things began to sour for us when we introduced our readers to the thinking of a molecular biologist named Peter Duesberg. Penned mostly by a writer named John Lauritsen, we gave extensive coverage to Duesberg's doubts about the HIV theory of AIDS. At first Duesberg was not sure what the cause of AIDS was, but he was certain it was not caused by a transmissible agent. As time went on, he began to promote a lifestyle theory of AIDS causation, pointing mainly to the use of recreational drugs.

Even though the scientific establishment did everything it could to debunk and silence Duesberg, he stood his ground and gained the support of a number of respected scientists and intellectuals who were also pilloried in one way or another for questioning the official AIDS dogma. I refer to his supporters and intellectuals who were inspired by him as "the Duesbergians." Even though there was a small army of Duesbergians, I have chosen to focus this book on four of the most prominent ones. Many of them had their own public and private theories about the causation of AIDS, but they generally had the same doubts about HIV as Duesberg. As the American government's official AIDS paradigm was increasingly carved into stone, Duesberg and the Duesbergians found themselves being called "AIDS denialists" who were a threat to public health. Some of the most powerful publications in the world mocked them, including *Science, Nature, The New York Times, The New York Review of Books,* and *The New Yorker.*

In addition to detailing Duesberg's critical thinking about the AIDS paradigm, John Lauritsen also reported on Duesberg's opposition to the use of some very toxic treatments for AIDS, most prominently, the drug called AZT which was being given to people who were diagnosed with AIDS or who had tested positive for HIV. Lauritsen's reporting on these matters are gathered in two important books, *The AIDS War,* and *Poison by Prescription.*

The *New York Native* became even more controversial in 1988 when I asked a writer, Neenyah Ostrom, to begin covering the relationship of AIDS to the mysterious emerging epidemic of what almost jokingly was called "chronic fatigue syndrome (CFS)." The obviously AIDS-like CFS epidemic had broken out concurrently with AIDS and seemed at first to mostly affect white heterosexual women. Ultimately, it was Ostrom's reporting in *New York Native* that was the biggest challenge to America's biomedical establishment, for it threatened to reveal that the entire AIDS paradigm was a house of cards and that the Centers for Disease Control was totally incompetent. Unfortunately for Duesberg and the Duesbegians, it also threatened to undermine the lifestyle paradigm of AIDS many of them were married to. Ostrom's reporting that AIDS and chronic fatigue syndrome were actually two faces of a large pandemic caused not by the retrovirus HIV but by HHV-6, a DNA virus that was able to infect and harm many systems in the body and seemed to cause variable illnesses. Her reporting supported the notion that the Centers for Disease Control had defined the AIDS epidemic *too narrowly*, and as a result they had made one of the biggest errors in the history of science and medicine. The HHV-6 theory of AIDS challenged everything about the epidemic: the nosology, the virology, the mode of transmission, and the epidemiology. It meant that at best HIV was an exponentially stupid mistake at best or, at worst, a nefarious cover-up.

The picture of an HHV-6 epidemic that could endanger the health of the entire public in a variety of ways was terrifying. Given that it is no secret that public health officials seem to consider "panic control" part of their job description, it really is not shocking that the Centers for Disease Control has foolishly tried to keep a lid on information about the HHV-6 pandemic for more than three decades.

I have been studying this cockamamie political and medical event for more than half of my 67 years on this planet. It has been the center of my adult life. I sometimes think of it as an existential Rubik's Cube that I needed to be able to figure out as completely as possible. I think Hannah Arendt felt the same way about the Holocaust and Nazi Germany and it inspired her to write *The Origins of Totalitarianism*. You could say that much of what I have been writing about the AIDS epidemic constitutes my attempt to come to grips with the origins of what I call "totalitarian science," "sociopathic science," or "abnormal science." Thomas Kuhn's discussion of "normal science" in *The Structure of Scientific Revolutions* inspired my opposite-world label "abnormal science" for the pseudoscience of AIDS and its related biomedical issues. Both Kuhn and Arendt have been for me what Arendt refers to as "bannisters" in my attempt to think my way through the moral, political, and scientific disaster that is Holocaust II.

Much of my thinking about Holocaust II is contained in my book, *Iatrogenocide: Notes for a Political Philosophy of Epidemiology and Science*. In the introduction to that book I write, "I have concluded that what we think of as the epidemiology and science of AIDS are essentially a corrupted hard drive. Virtually all science and epidemiology conducted on that hard drive is false even though it has the appearance of being rational, progressive, and normal."

I have also come to the conclusion that science is inherently political and the politics of AIDS science are both antigay and racist. Antigayness and racism are hardwired into the epidemiology and pseudoscience of AIDS in the same way that antisemitism was hardwired into Nazi science. I came up with the term "homodemiology" to describe the kind of antigay epidemiology and science that blames diseases and epidemics on gays and cherry-picks or distorts data to support unwarranted and bigoted conclusions. ("Afrodemiology" is my word for the racist version of the same concept.) In the so-called AIDS epidemic, "public health" is the mask that homodemiology and Afrodemiology wear.

In many ways, my journey to these conclusions began with Peter Duesberg and the Duesbergians. Peter Duesberg and his courageous colleagues spoke out when the science of AIDS contained elements that just didn't make sense. They all took great risks in speaking out and they inspired people like me to think critically about every element of the AIDS epidemic. Ironically, the more critically I thought about the epidemic the more I saw that the members of the AIDS establishment were not the only ones who were getting the epidemic wrong. As right as they were about some things, I came to the conclusion that Duesberg and the Duesbergians did not fully grasp the mistaken nosology and epidemiology or antigay politics of the epidemic. Furthermore, they did not see the massive epidemic of HHV-6 that was driving an apocalyptic and variable epidemic in plain sight—one that included chronic fatigue syndrome, autism, multiple sclerosis, and many other "mysterious" illnesses.

For the last three decades, Duesberg and Duesbergians have been sucking up all the oxygen in the AIDS debate. Their arguments about

HIV not being the cause of AIDS are cogent and it has been frustrating for them to watch the conventional wisdom triumph over truth. I think many of them are puzzled about their inability to wake up the intellectual community, the media, and the general public. I imagine many of them must lie in bed at night thinking "How can people be so stupid?"

I have written *Peter Duesberg and the Duesbergians* to celebrate their brilliance and bravery and to point out *what they got right*. I also discuss *what they got wrong* and explain why their mistakes prevented them from undermining a very corrupt AIDS establishment and thereby ending Holocaust II.

I hope they will accept my critique in the spirit of friendship and believe me when I say that, no matter what, I can never thank them enough for what they did. And what they almost did.

Half a Hero is Better than None

"As Max Weber put it, 'An exhaustive causal investigation of any concrete phenomenon in its full reality is not only impossible, it is simply nonsense.' Epidemiologists know this and do not attempt to include all causal factors in their analyses. They select some causes and omit others. Since the epidemiologist must, however, employ some criteria in the selection process, whether consciously or not, the final roundup of causes is never neutral. It necessarily reflects both the (human-made) rules of epidemiology and the values and assumptions of the person selecting the cause. The list probably reproduces many elements of the dominant political ideology as well, if only because the language we use to describe reality is so heavily influenced by the interests of powerful groups."
—Sylvia Noble Tesh, *Hidden Arguments: Political Ideology and Disease Prevention Policy* (Page 68)

To say that the achievement of Peter Duesberg is a glass half-full should never be seen as damning with faint praise. Unflappable, imperfect Peter Duesberg heroically changed the course of the AIDS epidemic and history itself by his actions and part of his personal tragedy is that he could have changed it even more if he had looked deeper and been more critically attentive to the politics of the Centers for Disease Control's heterosexist epidemiology.

In the introduction to his 1987 interview with Duesberg, John Lauritsen wrote, "Peter Duesberg came to the United States about 20 years ago from Germany. He is professor of Molecular Biology at the University of California in Berkeley. It is because of his interest in retroviruses, on which he is an authority, that he became involved in questioning the 'AIDS virus etiology.'" (*The Aids War* p.47)

In that interview Duesberg argued that HIV could not be the cause of AIDS because of "the consistent biochemical inactivity of the virus." (*AW* p.47) He told Lauritsen that "Even in patients who were dying from disease, the virus is almost undetectable, while RNA synthesis is essentially not detectable, (*AW* p.47) Duesberg also said, "So that is one of the key arguments, and there is no exception to the rule that pathogens in order to be pathogenic have to be active." (*AW* p.48) He insisted, "very few potentially susceptible cells are ever infected, and those that are infected don't do anything. The virus just sits here." (*AW* p.48)

Duesberg also argued that the long latency period of the disease was "a very suspicious signal that the virus is unlikely to be solely the direct cause as they claim." (AW p.48) He pointed out that retroviruses "are the most benign viruses that we know" and "they can remain in the cell in latent form." (*AW* p.49) And most damning of all to the HIV hypothesis, according to Duesberg, was the fact that "When AIDS is diagnosed, they say that now it's possible for the disease—but the virus is not doing any more than it had done before when there were no symptoms of the disease." (*AW* p.49) Duesberg concluded that the presence of antibodies to HIV was proof that the virus had been neutralized and asserted that it was "a gross injustice to discriminate against anyone on the basis of having antibodies." (*AW* p.50)

One of the most noble aspects of Duesberg's AIDS criticism and whistleblowing on the HIV mistake (or fraud) issue was his extraordinary—almost visionary—sensitivity to the damage it was going to do to the health and liberties of those who were victimized by it. In general, the people he argued with, those who benefited financially and professionally from the HIV hypothesis, had a rather cold and cavalier attitude toward the effect their brilliant ideas often had on the minorities who were affected. (They certainly never seemed to ask themselves what the consequences would be if *they* were wrong.)

Duesberg deserves credit for being one of the first people to realize (without saying as much) that the HIV/AIDS theory was an instance of what I've called "abnormal science." One of the wittiest men engaged in the AIDS issue, he could often find the humorous absurdities implicit in the HIV theory. When HIV was called a "slow virus," he said, "There are no slow viruses, only slow scientists." In public forums, he always presented his opinions in a collegial manner, but he was also always capable of leaving his opponents hemorrhaging from a cutting sarcasm presented with deadly charm. It may have been the fact that he verbally earned the role of the alpha intellect in any professional gathering that inspired both envy and vengeance from his powerful HIV establishment opponents. They were often simply intellectually outclassed, even if they held all the money and the political cards. Nothing rattles totalitarian science more than a clever and steadfast nontotalitarian scientist.

If Duesberg suffered from any deficits in the area of judgment, it may have been an inability to imagine a different AIDS epidemic caused by a dynamic, multisystemic virus like HHV-6 (and its family) which could manifest itself in a variety of surprising ways (like AIDS, chronic fatigue syndrome and autism) depending on other factors. Duesberg told Lauritsen, "AIDS is a condition which includes so many parameters that it's almost inconceivable to define a simple pathogen as the cause, considering the diverse patterns of the disease." (*AW* p.52) Duesberg didn't think outside the box of the CDC's nosology or epidemiology. He never considered the possibility that the CDC had missed a whole world of undetected nosological and epidemiological data (like the data from the chronic fatigue syndrome epidemic) that would have completely changed the picture of the disease's patterns. And the idea that there might be something in the world that could be called a multisystemic virus like HHV-6 which *could* cause many different patterns of disease, was simply not on his radar.

At the time that Lauritsen first interviewed Duesberg—in 1987— Duesberg remained a bit of an agnostic on what was actually causing AIDS, saying, "We haven't excluded anything" and "I really wonder what it could be." (*AW* p.53) Compared to where he would end up, he was a demure etiological virgin at that point. He was only beginning to consider the role of recreational drugs as a possible cause saying, "I'm really just guessing here, but I think this is where more research should be done." (*AW* p.53)

Unfortunately, as time went on Duesberg seems to have been encouraged or even pressured by some of his colleagues to take a stronger public stand on what he thought actually *was* the cause of AIDS and he became far less tentative and open-minded, passionately adding to his anti-HIV gospel a seemingly unshakable conviction that recreational drugs explained AIDS in gay men. Regardless of its merits, such a position immediately lost him the readymade constituency of the gay community who seemed to have been invited by Duesberg and his followers to be exonerated for a transmissible infection only to be convicted as a group in an alternative fashion for having a unique gay (and—let's not forget—criminal) drug-taking lifestyle. With some notable exceptions, Duesberg walked into a big gay "thanks but no thanks." He had jumped the gay shark. It was a tragic development for both parties, because politically, Duesberg really needed gay supporters to help him challenge the mistaken HIV hypothesis, which he felt was unfairly threatening their liberties and health of the gay community. He was the enemy of the gay community's determined CDC/NIH enemy, but he wasn't perceived as its friend. By rejecting Duesberg's half-a-glass of truth about the virus, the gay community ended up in the open arms of the AIDS establishment and crusading public health authorities complete with all the goodies they had in store for their willing, eager and all too compliant patient population.

Peter Duesberg detailed his argument about the nature of the AIDS epidemic and his struggle with the AIDS establishment in his book, *Inventing the AIDS Virus*, which was published by Regnery Publishing in 1998. In the publisher's preface, Alfred Regnery notes, "AIDS is the first political disease." In his acknowledgments, Duesberg wrote, "I extend my gratitude to my most critical opponents in the AIDS debate, who have unwittingly provided me the great volume of evidence by which I have disproved the virus-AIDS hypothesis and exposed the political maneuverings behind the war on AIDS." (*IAV* p.x)

Duesberg's book could be used as a primary text if college courses are ever given on the politics, sociology and psychology of what I call "abnormal science." He fleshes out many parts of his argument against the HIV theory of AIDS causation already mentioned in his 1987 interview with Lauritsen. While Duesberg is often thought to be someone who encouraged the rethinking of the AIDS issue, the book supports the notion already mentioned that, in reality, he actually *never went far enough*, never really did a true radical rethinking of AIDS because he works with a tacit acceptance of the basic epidemiological premises and "facts" provided by the CDC and the HIV/AIDS establishment. By leaving their paradigm's "factual" assumptions standing, he ultimately jeopardized his own analysis. Duesberg's critical tact was to take the "facts" as they were provided by the CDC and to try and poke holes in their etiological logic by showing how they failed to successfully make predictions about the course of the epidemic or by arguing that the facts as given by the CDC contradicted other formally known (hence, published) facts. The problem was that AIDS involved ground zero nosological and epidemiological definitions of what an AIDS case actually was, and *if* that definition had, at the very beginning of the epidemic, been distorted by evidence that had been cherry-picked, or had been ignored because of political blinders, then there was a good chance that Duesberg—even with his superb skills of logic and reason—was trapped in an pseudoscientific funhouse of "garbage in garbage out." Saying the CDC mistakenly linked the wrong virus to cases of AIDS begs a question: And what if the CDC completely got the definition of AIDS cases wrong to begin with? Or, more troubling, that what the CDC thought were epidemiological apples and oranges were really all apples or all oranges? Duesberg never illuminated *all* of the fundamental possibilities of what could have gone wrong nosologically and epidemiologically. Duesberg was in a Donald Rumsfeld situation where he didn't know what he didn't know.

Duesberg worked with the epidemiological predictions the AIDS authorities were giving him and tried to show that when the predictions based on them did not work out, they reflected poorly on the credibility of the HIV theory. He argued, "Officials have continually predicted the explosion of AIDS into the general population through sexual transmission of HIV, striking males and females equally, as well as homosexuals and heterosexuals, to be followed by a corresponding increase in the rate of death. . . . In short, the alleged viral disease does not seem to be spreading from the 1 million HIV-positive Americans to the remaining 250 million." (*IAV* p.5)

Duesberg's logic brilliantly skewered the CDC's notion that AIDS was an equal opportunity disease. But again, one has to note that the one caveat he didn't acknowledge was that if the CDC's definition of what an AIDS case was *turned out to be dead wrong*, then all bets were off about correlated and potentially causative factors. Just debunking the logic behind the weak correlation of putative AIDS cases with HIV was not the same as debunking the notion of *some fundamentally different kind of AIDS epidemic* still occurring, not only in the gay community, but also in some form in the general population. If, at the very basic level of defining what a case is and what a case isn't, profound mistakes had been made, then one couldn't really know where the disease was and where it wasn't. And then the issue of HIV not being the cause of what was being called AIDS would, in that case, be *totally beside the point*. If anything, the HIV mistake should have made people wonder if those in charge at the CDC had gotten something even more profoundly wrong in the initial working definition of AIDS which subsequently was carved in stone thanks to the totalitarian scientific culture that protected it.

Insofar as Duesberg recognized that it all just didn't add up, he graciously performed a great humanitarian service over and over again by telling the world that as long as the HIV establishment was in charge of AIDS we were essentially trapped in a realm of unreliable and untrustworthy pseudoscience where people were going to get hurt. And luckily, for three decades, at great personal expense, Duesberg valiantly refused to shut up. Perplexed, Duesberg wrote, "Something is wrong with this picture. How could the largest and most sophisticated scientific establishment in history have failed so miserably in saving lives and even in forecasting the epidemic's toll?" (*IAV* p.5) Ironically, given that Duesberg himself was blind to what turned out to be the CFS epidemic and HHV-6 spectrum catastrophe, the premise of his rhetorical question turned out to be a tragic understatement.

Duesberg's suggestion about what should be done reinforces the notion that his call to a reassessment of AIDS and HIV just wasn't intellectually radical or fundamental enough. Duesberg's prescription for the problem was that "Faced with this medical debacle, scientists should re-open a simple but most essential question: What causes AIDS?" (*IAV* p.6) Again, it was not really a radical return to epidemiological ground zero. A return to ground zero would have involved asking if the epidemiological common immunological denominator that determined what a case actually was itself needed to be audited by looking closely—and in an immunologically sophisticated manner—*at the entire population*. Duesberg was like an accountant who looks at the books for discrepancies, but never goes into the warehouse to see if what's there matches the inventory numbers. His due diligence only went so far. The definition of AIDS was on the books and unfortunately, taken at face value by Duesberg. It didn't necessarily match what was actually going on in doctor's offices all over America and it didn't necessarily reflect the actual disaster that was occurring in the immune systems of the entire American population. There was a whole immunologically-challenged world beyond the CDC's published data and the peer-reviewed papers Duesberg used to play "gotcha" with the CDC's facts, logic, and conclusions.

There was an interesting groupthink bias in Duesberg and many of his followers, most of whom were heterosexual—some emphatically so. Not surprisingly, their notion about what was wrong with AIDS etiology *was always biased in the direction of heterosexuals being less (or not at all) at risk for AIDS* as a result of the CDC's scientific errors. Sometimes one got the uncanny notion that Duesberg and his followers were whistling heterosexually in the dark, engaged in trying to convince themselves that *they as a group* were safe from the "gay lifestyle" epidemic. Ironically, considering their apparent need for personal immunological safety, though, is the fact that *if* the CDC was wrong then all bets about their safety could have been off and the actual level of risk could have gone the other way. *They could have been in more, not less danger.* But that possibility never seemed to consciously dawn on them, and their AIDS dissident movement, in all its forms, seemed bent on making sure that it never did. They created a kind of dissident groupthink that made them odd bedfellows with the mostly white male heterosexual HIV establishment who also could absolutely not let themselves see the connection between AIDS, chronic fatigue syndrome, HHV-6, and ultimately the simmering HHV-6-related autism disaster.

Duesberg got a lot of things right and a lot of things sort of right. He was right when he wrote that "Without going back to check its underlying assumptions, the AIDS establishment will never make sense of its mountain of data." (*IAV* p.6) He didn't quite get it right when he concluded, "The single flaw that determined the destiny of AIDS research since 1984 was the assumption that AIDS is infectious. After taking this wrong turn scientists had to make bad assumptions upon which they have built a huge artifice of mistaken ideas." (*IAV* p.6) Duesberg very simply failed to notice the fundamental wrong turn that was made before *that* wrong turn. He never considered the possibility that if the definition of AIDS itself was wrong, the corrected definition just might support the notion of an infectious epidemic and a virus-AIDS hypothesis, *just not the mistaken HIV one.*

The great thing about Duesberg—for students of what I've called homodemiology or heterosexist epidemiology—is that he criticized the logical absurdity of what I call GRID-think, (Gay-related immune deficiency) which is in part the rather superstitious and bigoted notion implicit in HIV epidemiology that *viruses know intuitively who gays are* so they can choose to infect them and only them. Unfortunately, Duesberg built his own quasi-GRID-think drug-and-lifestyle-paradigm on a similar reality-challenged premise by saying that something non-infectious must explain an epidemic confining itself mainly to a risk group. By pointing out the logical absurdity of a virus limiting itself to one group of people, he opened the way for a more radical critical political rethinking about what was going on in the CDC's epidemiology that he seemed unprepared to do himself. He started the job, but homodemiological and sociological analysis had to finish it. Blaming lifestyle factors of gays was just another not-very-great correlation fingered as causation, generating an alternative scapegoating epidemiology of blaming the victims for what turned out to be the HHV-6 spectrum catastrophe. Unfortunately, Duesberg exposed one wild goose chase and started another one when he wrote, "The only solution is to rethink the basic assumption that AIDS is infectious and is caused by HIV." (*IAV* p.7) The only solution? Well, not exactly.

Duesberg's book will always be an important source for anyone who wants to understand the evolution of the AIDS mistake, even if Duesberg's own theory turned out to be wrong. Most importantly,

Duesberg details just how abnormal and nearly psychotic the whole scientific process of AIDS was and his work supports the argument that something with a totalitarian *je ne sais quoi* was unfolding in the name of AIDS science.

The very manner in which HIV was announced in 1984 as the probable cause of AIDS, according to Duesberg's account, was scientifically deviant: "This announcement was made prior to the publication of any scientific evidence confirming the virus theory. With this unprecedented maneuver, Gallo's discovery bypassed review by the scientific community. Science by press conference was substituted for the unconventional process of scientific validation, which is based on publications in the professional literature. The 'AIDS virus' became instant national dogma, and the tremendous weight of federal resources were diverted into just one race—the race to study the AIDS virus . . . . The only questions to be studied from 1984 on were how HIV causes AIDS and what could be done about it." (*IAV* p.8)

At that point in time, Duesberg noted that "serious doubts are now surfacing about HIV, the so-called AIDS virus . . . . . The consensus on the virus hypothesis of AIDS is falling apart, as its opponents grow in number." (*IAV* p.8) At that moment Duesberg still seemed optimistic, as AIDS seemed to be taking place in the good faith universe of normal science which was open to change and paradigm shift. Unfortunately, because he was blind to the heterosexist sociological issues underpinning AIDS, he was incapable of perceiving the unmovable backstage anti-gay epidemiological values that were controlling the public health agenda and polluting the science. He couldn't see that it wasn't just a matter of the practitioners of this deviant science were digging in professionally; the whole homodemiological culture was dug in, which was far more formidable than anything Duesberg could have imagined. The political consensus about the etiological nature of "AIDS" was not a just stone in the road of scientific process. Peter Duesberg had found his way into abnormal science's opposite world.

As a paradigm that was supposed to capture people's imagination and cause a major shift or Kuhnian conversion—or visual gestalt-shift—from one consensus to another, Duesberg's paradigm was nearly dead on arrival. If he had simply taken his stand as a dean of retrovirology and just left the cause of AIDS up in the air and concentrated on demolishing the HIV theory once and for all, the HHV-6 catastrophe and what I call "Holocaust II" might have been stopped in their tracks.

Duesberg charged that the CDC's paradigm was "ineffective" and that "public fear was being exploited." (*IAV* p. 9) From his perspective, the public was being told the problem was bigger than it actually was. True, public fear was being shamelessly exploited, but *not in the way Duesberg thought.* By framing the epidemic in an anti-gay manner, public fear of gays, society's sexual outsiders, *was* being manipulated to hide the painful truth about the public's risk of developing a complex form of immunodeficiency or dysfunction. The public was being provided with what Daniel Goleman called "a vital lie." A terrified public, to the great detriment of its future health was getting the reassuring heterosexist pseudo-facts about "AIDS" it wanted to hear with the gay community losing what I call its *epidemiological human rights* in the process. And again, ironically, Duesberg and the Duesbergians had their own set of heterosexist concoctions that were *even more reassuring* to the heterosexual general population. And wrong. Both the CDC paradigm and the Duesberg paradigm misled a clueless and anxious public.

Duesberg's shock at the nature of what was going on is exactly why a formal theory of abnormal or totalitarian science is required to comprehend and illuminate the AIDS era, just as the concept of totalitarianism was required to understand the Hitler and Stalin eras. Duesberg asks a big, ugly, rhetorical question: "How could a whole new generation of more than a hundred thousand AIDS experts, including medical doctors, virologists, immunologists, cancer researchers, pharmacologists, and epidemiologists—including more than half a dozen Nobel Laureates—be wrong? How could a scientific world that so freely exchanged all information from every corner of this planet have missed an alternative explanation for AIDS?" (*IAV* p.9) Too bad he didn't ask how the exact same crowd could not see the chronic fatigue syndrome epidemic for what it was. Ditto for HHV-6 and its insidious spectrum.

Again, Duesberg's answer to his own question was that AIDS had been misclassified as an infectious illness and his theory rested on the notion that "the premature assumption of contagiousness has many times in the past obstructed free investigation for the treatment and prevention of a non-infectious disease—sometimes for years, at the cost of many thousands of lives." (*LAV* p.10) Duesberg was setting the terms of the twenty-five-year debate between the mainstream AIDS establishment and what became popularly known as the AIDS dissidents, or the Duesbergians. This unfortunate dichotomy set the course for the wrong kind of debate, a contest between HIV and Duesberg's non-infectious drug lifestyle hypothesis, leaving out the possibility that there might be a dynamic infectious agent *other than HIV* that did indeed fit the causation criteria of a redefined AIDS epidemic. No space was left in the debate for something like a new multisystemic virus such as HHV-6, which was capable of causing an epidemic of a more broadly defined variable illness. Duesberg asserted HIV "could be the most harmful of . . . fatal errors in the history of medicine if AIDS proves to be not infectious." (*LAV* p.10) Of course, if AIDS was incorrectly defined and a dynamic viral agent other than HIV was spreading *silently and exponentially* while the false Duesbergian debate sucked up all of intellectual and scientific oxygen in the debate on AIDS, the harm could have been exponentially worse. And it was.

In order for abnormal or totalitarian science to hold sway over a society for a long period of time, it must have ample cooperation from both the scientific and media communities and the Duesberg story provides evidence that such was the case in AIDS. To explain how the media was continuously kept in its subservient place during the AIDS debacle, he quotes reporter Elinor Burkett of *The Miami Herald*: "If you have an AIDS beat, you're a beat reporter, your job is every day to go out there, fill your newspaper with what's new about AIDS. You write a story that questions the truth of the central AIDS hypothesis and what happened to me will happen to you. Nobody's going to talk to you. Now if nobody will talk to you, if nobody at the CDC will ever return your phone call, you lose your competitive edge as an AIDS reporter. So it always keeps you in the mainstream, because you need those guys to be your buddies . . . ." (*LAV* p.388)

Duesberg insists that the very defensive and insular AIDS scientific establishment was determined to "confine the debate to scientific circles." (*IAV* p.389) He quotes a rather shocking threat from the de facto AIDS Czar, Anthony Fauci, who said, "Journalists who make too many mistakes, or who are sloppy are going to find that their access to scientists may diminish."(*IAV* p.384) In a totalitarian world of homodemiology and abnormal science the definition of "sloppy" will be that which contradicts the powers that be. Question AIDS and you will need to look for a new career. (Given the degree to which AIDS science often looks like a big unmade bed, it's amusing to hear Fauci say the word "sloppy" with a straight face.)

Duesberg also quotes two of the powerful, public-relations-savvy virologists who suggested another tactic for dealing with Duesberg and the critics of the HIV establishment: "One approach would be to refuse television confrontations with Duesberg, as Tony Fauci and one of us managed to do at the opening of the VIIth International Conference on AIDS in Florence. One can't spread misinformation without an audience." (*IAV* p.39) There's nothing in Thomas Kuhn's theories about the process of normal science about deliberately denying one's critics an audience, or denying the public exposure to scientific second and third opinions.

One of the more outrageous moments in his book occurs when Duesberg writes, "Based on an anonymous source, key officials of the United States government specifically engineered a strategy for suppressing the HIV debate in 1987 while Duesberg was still on leave at the N.I.H. The operation began on April 28, less than a month after Duesberg's first paper on the HIV question appeared in *Cancer Research*, apparently because several journalists and homosexual activists began raising questions." (*IAV* p.32) A memo about Duesberg's critique of the HIV theory was sent out from a staffer in the Office of the Secretary of Health and Human Services: "This obviously has the potential to raise a lot of controversy (If this isn't the virus, how do we know the blood supply is safe? How do we know anything about transmission? How could you all be so stupid, and why should we ever believe you again?) And we need to be prepared to respond. I have already asked N.I.H. public affairs to start digging into this." (*IAV* p.390) This is an extremely important memo from the point of view of future what-did-they-know-and-when-did-they-know-it histories that try to fathom all the government's motivations throughout this scientific and political disaster. It shows how clearly at least one person in the government could see the potential dire consequences for the government of being wrong about HIV. Somebody knew *exactly* what was at stake.

In his book, Duesberg gives a number of examples of the media seeming to have been pressured by the HIV establishment *not to cover the story of the controversy*. According to Duesberg, "The MacNeil Lehrer News hour sent camera crews to do a major segment on the controversy. But when the . . . broadcast date arrived, the feature had been pulled. Apparently AIDS officials had heard of its imminent airing and had intercepted it." (*IAV* p.392) Television shows on Duesberg involving Good Morning America on ABC, CNN, Italian television, and Larry King Live met with a similar fate.

According to Duesberg's book, he "appeared on major national television only twice. The first time was on March 28, 1993 on the ABC magazine program *Day One*. Even in this case, according to the producer, Fauci tried to get the show canceled days before broadcast.' (*IAV* p.393) When Duesberg was interviewed for *Nightline*, he ended up only being given a small amount of air time and Fauci showed up and was given the lion's share of the show to make the HIV establishment's case. And Duesberg fared no better overseas. The British medical and public health establishment greeted a pro-Duesberg program with "stern condemnations" and subsequently the British press "turned around and began criticizing the program." (*IAV* p.323)

One of the most interesting moments of censorship occurred at the highest level of government when "Jim Warner, a Reagan White House advisor critical of AIDS alarmism, heard about Duesberg and arranged a White House debate in January 1988." (*IAV* p.394) Duesberg writes, "This would have forced the HIV issue into the public spotlight, but it was abruptly canceled days ahead of time, on orders from above." (*IAV* p.394)

Duesberg didn't fare much better with the print media. He notes that *The New York Times* had written about him only three times in the first seven years of the controversy and all of it was negative. The same kind of treatment was doled out by *The Washington Post* and "the *San Francisco Chronicle* intended to cover the story, until it encountered opposition from scientists in the local AIDS establishment." (*IAV* p.394) Even the countercultural or alternative press could not be counted on to give the controversy balanced or independent-minded coverage. Duesberg reports, "In 1989 *Rolling Stone* had commissioned a freelance writer from New York to write a Duesberg article, but then canceled it during the interview with Duesberg in his lab." (*IAV* p.395) Both *Harper's* and *Esquire* killed articles that had been commissioned on Duesberg during the same period. The media was essentially acting as an enabler of the culture of abnormal or totalitarian science.

Even more evidence that AIDS was a manifestation of abnormal science can be found in the way that Duesberg experienced censorship from formerly adoring scientific circles and experienced roadblocks to having his ideas and criticisms presented in the professional scientific literature. Duesberg writes, "Robert Gallo and some other scientists began refusing . . . to attend scientific conferences if Duesberg would be allowed to make a presentation." (*IAV* p.396) During the same period Duesberg rarely was "invited to retrovirus meetings and virtually never to AIDS conferences, despite seminal contributions to the field, including the isolation of the retroviral genome, the first analysis of the order of retroviral genes, and the discovery of the first retroviral cancer gene." (*IAV* p.396)

Duesberg reports that his scientific papers on AIDS "would constantly run into obstacles at every turn, from hostile peer reviews to reluctant editors."(*IAV* p.393) The rules mysteriously changed for "the *Proceedings of the National Academy of Sciences*, where Academy members such as Duesberg have an automatic right to publish papers without standard peer review." (*IAV* p.397) An editor rejected Duesberg's unique and provocative submission by bizarrely saying that it was not "original." And, supporting the case for the arbitrary make-it-up-as-you-go-along nature of abnormal AIDS science, a subsequent replacement editor decided tradition had to be completely ignored for this special case and the Duesberg paper had to be peer-reviewed *because it was "controversial."* (*IAV* p.397) It took several months of hostile reviewers negotiating with Duesberg before the paper was finally published. According to Duesberg, "Robert Gallo was asked to write a rebuttal, but never did." (*IAV* p.357) Strategic silent treatment is part of the arsenal of abnormal science.

The punishments for anyone standing up to totalitarian, abnormal science can be severe. Duesberg reports that "the AIDS establishment made its most effective counterattack by going after Duesberg's funding, the lifeblood of any scientist's laboratory. After coming out against the HIV theory, Duesberg was denied continuation of an N.I.H. Outstanding Grant by a group of scientists which included two who were proponents of the HIV paradigm and three scientists who never even reviewed the grant. When a review committee considered Duesberg's grant proposal a few months later, "they did . . . complain about Duesberg's questioning attitude as the major obstacle to funding him and singled out AIDS." (*IAV* p.402) Subsequently, "every one of his seventeen peer-reviewed grant applications to other federal state or private agencies—whether for AIDS research, on AZT and other drugs, or for cancer research—has been turned down." (*IAV* p.403) Thus did Duesberg come face to face with one of the telltale signs of abnormal and totalitarian science: blacklisting. The long arms of HIV/AIDS politics reached into his life at his university where "Several fellow professors" maneuvered "against Duesberg in various ways." His promotions in pay were "blocked" and he was denied "coveted graduate lecture courses." (*IAV* p.404)

One of the most dramatic and creepiest abnormal science moments in the Duesberg saga occurred in 1994 when a high-ranking geneticist from the N.I.H. flew to California to present Duesberg with an unpublished paper titled "HIV Causes AIDS: Koch's Postulates Fulfilled." Duesberg was asked to be a third author on a paper *he hadn't even collaborated on.* The paper had been commissioned by *Nature* editor and HIV theory proponent, John Maddox. Duesberg was warned by his high-ranking visitor that by continuing his opposition to the HIV theory he "would even risk his credentials for having discovered cancer genes." (*IAV* p.406) (The willingness to "disappear" the past is another one of the telltale signs of totalitarian science.) The geneticist told Duesberg that if he agreed to be an author on the paper it would "open the doors for Duesberg's reentry into the establishment." (*IAV* p 406) Duesberg said thanks but no thanks in the form of offering to write something for *Nature* that said the direct opposite of what that proposed unsigned paper posited.

A very thoughtful and philosophical man in many ways, Duesberg sought to understand the recalcitrant system that was making it so difficult for his ideas to be heard and tested, let alone prevail. He blamed it on "command science" which by his analysis, derived its power from three sources in the medical establishment: "(1) enforced consensus through peer review, (2) enforced consensus through commercialization and (3) the fear of disease, particularly infectious disease." (*IAV* p.452)

Because all serious medical scientists in America need grants from the NIH to survive, they often need to conform to the establishment viewpoint. While the "peer-review system" is supposed to be like an independent jury system, in reality, according to Duesberg, "a truly independent jury system would be fatal to the establishment." (*IAV* p.452) The result is "the peers serve the orthodoxy by serving their own vested interests." (*IAV* p.452) Duesberg warned that "as long as a scientist's work is reviewed only by competitors within his own field, peer review will crush genuine science." (*IAV* p.454)

Ominously for AIDS patients and the myriad victims of the real AIDS epidemic, Duesberg concluded that "Through peer review the federal government has attained a near-monopoly on science." (*IAV* p.454) Abnormal science loves the absolute power of monopolies. HIV became hegemonic because "a handful of federal agencies, primarily the NIH, dominate research policies and effectively dictate the official dogma . . . . By declaring the virus the cause of AIDS at a press conference sponsored by the Department of Health and Human Services, NIH researcher Robert Gallo swung the entire medical establishment and even the rest of the world, behind his hypothesis. Once such a definitive statement is made, the difficulty of retracting it only increases with time."(*IAV* p.454)

Duesberg criticized the huge conflict of interest in science that is caused by its commercialization. He argued that the FDA, by essentially banning competing therapies, often helps the pharmaceutical industry develop monopolies. Profits from products approved by the FDA often find their way back to scientists who sat in judgment on fellow scientists "in the form of patent royalties, consultantships, paid board positions, and stock ownership." (*IAV* p.455) In addition, "in order for a research product to find a market, the underlying hypothesis for the product must be accepted by a majority of the practitioners in the field." (*IAV* p.455) In the case of AIDS "commercial success can be achieved only by consensus. For example, an AIDS hypothesis would not be approved unless it miraculously cured AIDS overnight." (*IAV* p.455) Thus Gallo's royalties from an HIV patent as well as those with financial interest in HIV tests (Like William Haseltine and Max Essex) indicate that they may not be the most disinterested parties to make important decisions about the direction of AIDS research. And yet they were among the powerful inner circle of AIDS research. No wonder Duesberg often experienced forms of petulance and hostility from such characters rather than open-minded collegiality. In essence, by telling an inconvenient truth he was a threat to their lifestyles and reputations.

The third arm of the "command science" which Duesberg discusses goes in the opposite direction of the overriding conclusion of my newspaper's reporting about the real AIDS epidemic. Duesberg writes, "Traditionally, the power of medical science has been based on the fear of disease, particularly infectious disease. The HIV-AIDS establishment has exploited this instrument of power to its limit." (*IAV* p.456) Duesberg assumes that an infectious epidemic has essentially been invented out of whole cloth by incompetent epidemiology. His book would have been more accurately titled "Inventing the AIDS Epidemic." Duesberg accuses the CDC of delusional epidemiology driven by opportunism and hysteria. The manipulated paradigm of an infectious AIDS epidemic was used to create a "stampede," to create "irrational" fear in the public, to cynically manipulate, to mislead. And most importantly, from the Duesberg perspective, to build a lucrative new empire for the CDC.

While most of my work which began at *New York Native* supports the notion of a reign of intellectual dishonesty at the CDC, my conclusions about AIDS turn this part of the Duesbergian thesis on its head. Duesberg sees a devastating, apocalyptic epidemic being cynically and opportunistically *imagined*, and my reporting sees it as *existing—big time—and being concealed*. Other than HIV not being the cause of AIDS, the only thing Duesberg and I fundamentally agree on (in addition to the questionable behavior of many powerful individuals) is that the AIDS establishment was not really doing science as we expect it to be done. Duesberg might even agree with the premise that the science of AIDS was abnormal, totalitarian and even psychotic.

There is one other thing that Duesberg got right that deserves special mention. Duesberg performed an heroic whistle-blowing act during dark hours of the epidemic: his fearless adoption of a principled stand against the administration of AZT to AIDS patients. In a chapter of his book aptly titled, "With Therapies Like this, Who Needs Disease?", he discussed Azidothymidine, or AZT. About this very toxic drug that was being given to AIDS patients, Duesberg writes, "AZT kills dividing cells anywhere in the body—causing ulcerations and hemorrhaging; damage to hair follicles and skin; killing mitochondria, the energy cells of the brain; wasting away of muscles; and the destruction of the immune system and other cells. . . . Amazingly, AZT was first approved for treatment of AIDS in 1987 and then for prevention of AIDS in 1990." (*IAV* p.301) Duesberg didn't say it, but he didn't have to. AZT was more of a cruel, sadistic, toxic punishment than a medical treatment for AIDS patients.

AZT beautifully expressed the AIDS zeitgeist. AZT was invented in 1964 to kill cancer tumors, but the drug also effectively killed healthy growing tissues and was shelved without a patent because it was too toxic. Twenty years later scientists reported that it was capable of stopping HIV from replicating. Duesberg had serious doubts about even the basic AIDS research that was done with AZT which suggested that it could be given in small enough doses so that it would kill the virus without also killing the t-cells and other cells in the body. Not surprisingly, given the nature of AIDS science, the research that supported the safety of using AZT could not be subsequently replicated and showed that "the same low concentration [of AZT] that stops HIV also kills cells." (*IAV* p.313) Like much of the abnormal science of AIDS, if you looked diligently beneath one fraud, you could find yet another.

The person most responsible for foisting this quasi-genocidal toxic drug on AIDS patients was Sam Broder, the man who was Gallo's boss at the National Cancer Institute. He was the man responsible for the original questionable research suggesting that AZT could be given in doses that wouldn't harm patients. AIDS patients would pay a horrifying price for his scientific slovenliness. Duesberg notes, "Broder and his collaborators have never corrected their original reports, nor have they explained the huge discrepancies between their data and other reports." (*IAV* p.313)

Duesberg's critique of AZT gets even more devastating when he points out that the virus is dormant and therefore the virus "can only attack growing cells" and "like all other chemotherapeutic drugs, is unable to distinguish an HIV-infected cell from one that is uninfected. This has disastrous consequences on AZT-treated people; since only 1 in about 500 t-cells of HIV anti-body positive persons is ever infected, AZT must kill 499 good t-cells to kill just one that is infected by the hypothetical AIDS virus." (*IAV* p.313) In a sardonic understatement, Duesberg concluded, "It is a tragedy for people who already suffer from a t-cell deficiency." (*IAV* p.314) Needless to say, as time passes, giving people AZT sounds more and more unquestionably like a form of genocidal insanity or what I call "iatrogenocide." For a few who watched in horror as this transpired, it did *then*, too. Duesberg wrote "A toxic chemotherapy was about to be unleashed on AIDS victims, but no one had the time to think twice about its potential to destroy the immune systems of people who might otherwise survive." (*IAV* p.314) AZT belonged more in a court room as Exhibit A of a crimes against humanity trial than in the bodies of AIDS patients.

Unfortunately, given all the surreal terror and hysteria of the time and the prevalent abject mentality of the patients, the gay community and its doctors wanted something—virtually anything—that could (or seemed to) address the problem. But make no mistake about it. There were also financial considerations that helped create the AZT disaster. Burroughs Welcome, the company that owned the patent on the drug, was eager to win approval for the treatment of AIDS by the FDA. Unfortunately for the AIDS patients, Burroughs Welcome's head researcher worked closely and effectively with Sam Broder to get FDA approval.

The process of testing the effectiveness of the drug was also highly questionable. The double blind, placebo-controlled studies of AZT on AIDS patients were not exactly double blind and placebo controlled. They were as abnormal as just about everything else in the Kafkaesque world of AIDS science. The list of things that went off the rails in the study was long. The study was stopped prematurely because the positive "results seemed stupendous." (*IAV* p.316) But as scientists looked more closely at the details of the study it turned out that the AZT trial was just as unreliable as much of the basic laboratory science that had launched AZT in the first place. More placebo patients had died than seemed reasonable. A close look at the study revealed that many of the AZT users had suffered horrific side effects which were downplayed even though they "more than abolished its presumed benefit." (*IAV* p.317)

When more information surfaced about the AZT trial, it turned out that the controls for the study were a complete mess. It was virtually impossible to conceal which patients were on AZT because in patients on AZT the drug killed bone marrow cells so quickly, that patients would come down with aplastic anemia, a not-hard-to-detect dreadful disease. According to Duesberg, "the patients, needless to say, often found out what they were taking" (*IAV* p.318) from clues like throwing up blood or changes in their blood counts. That had a grimly ironic effect on the study because those who discovered they were on the placebo, by comparing the tastes of their pills with the pills of those who were actually taking AZT, *wanted to take what they had been told was the life saving AZT.* It was a heartbreaking sign of the desperation and helplessness of their situation. According to Duesberg, "the patients had bought the early rumors of AZT's incredible healing powers, and they really did not want to take a placebo. Some of the placebo group secretly did use AZT, explaining the presence of its toxic side effects among those patients." (*IAV* p.318)

Because doctors easily noticed in the so-called "blinded" study that the AZT patients *seemed* to be doing better than the non-AZT patients, the study was ended early. The study's credibility was in shambles when it turned out that some of the patients on AZT had to be taken off of it because it was so toxic. According to Duesberg, "many of the patients simply could not tolerate AZT, and the physicians had to do something to save their lives." (*IAV* p.319) And "15 percent of the AZT group disappeared, possibly including patients with the most severe side effects." (*IAV* p.319) An inspection of documents pertaining to the study obtained under the Freedom of Information Act revealed a wide array of abnormalities in the study that suggested the study was one of the more notable frauds of the AIDS Era and Holocaust II.

While the initial results of the AZT study indicated an improvement of t-cells, it turned out that a temporary increase of t-cells did not really indicate that the patients were getting better. And there might have been some improvement of the patients from a broad spectrum antibiotic effect. The only problem was that *the drug was also toxically undermining the immune system*. It was opposite world science at its best. AZT was in essence becoming another cause of AIDS.

Tragically, even though the study was a scientific train wreck, the FDA approved AZT. The FDA panel that approved AZT included two paid consultants from Burroughs Wellcome. Duesberg notes, "the FDA endorsement could seem a cruel joke perpetrated by heartless AIDS scientists. Patients on AZT receive little more than white capsules surrounded by a blue band. But every time lab researchers order another batch for experimentation they receive a special label . . . A skull-and-crossbones symbol appears on background of bright orange, signifying an unusual chemical hazard." (*IAV* p.324)